PRAISE FOR *Orga*

"I have been a natural health care provider for over 35 years. Hippocrates said "Our food should be our medicine". In the 15 years that I've known Beverly she has never wavered from her passion for educating people in the importance of eating nutritious and healthy foods prepared correctly. This book of delightful recipes validates that passion. It is truly gratifying to find a book that focuses on foods that nourish our bodies in a healthful way and tastes good too."

— KATHLEEN I. GREGG, ND, PhD
Director, Health Matters, Inc.
drgregg@healthmattersmi.com

"*Organize Eating: A Cookbook for Transitioning to Plant-Based Meals* is right on time as more people look for information and resources to help them adopt healthier lifestyles. The techniques and recipes Beverly has developed will help you to get better organized so you can progress more confidently along your healthy eating journey."

— AKUA WOOLBRIGHT, PhD
National Nutrition Program Director
Whole Cities Foundation

"Drawing on over thirty years of experience, Beverly Flemings' Organize Eating Cookbook contains all you need to know about transitioning to a plant-based seasonal diet. Beverly's advice on everything from choosing seasonal foods, organizing your kitchen, and preparing healthful dishes makes this an invaluable guide to modern day living."

— DON CINZORI,
pioneer & organic vegetable farmer
Cinzori Family Farm - Ceresco, MI
Certified Organic since 1985
www.cinzorifarms.com

"After decades of experience with healthy eating, Beverly has created a practical and relatable food guide that will benefit many!"

— ERIN BEATTIE, RDN
Registered Dietitian Nutritionist
Founder of Thriving Health, LLC

Organize Eating

To your health
Live long, live strong!.
Blessings!
Beverly 8/11/22

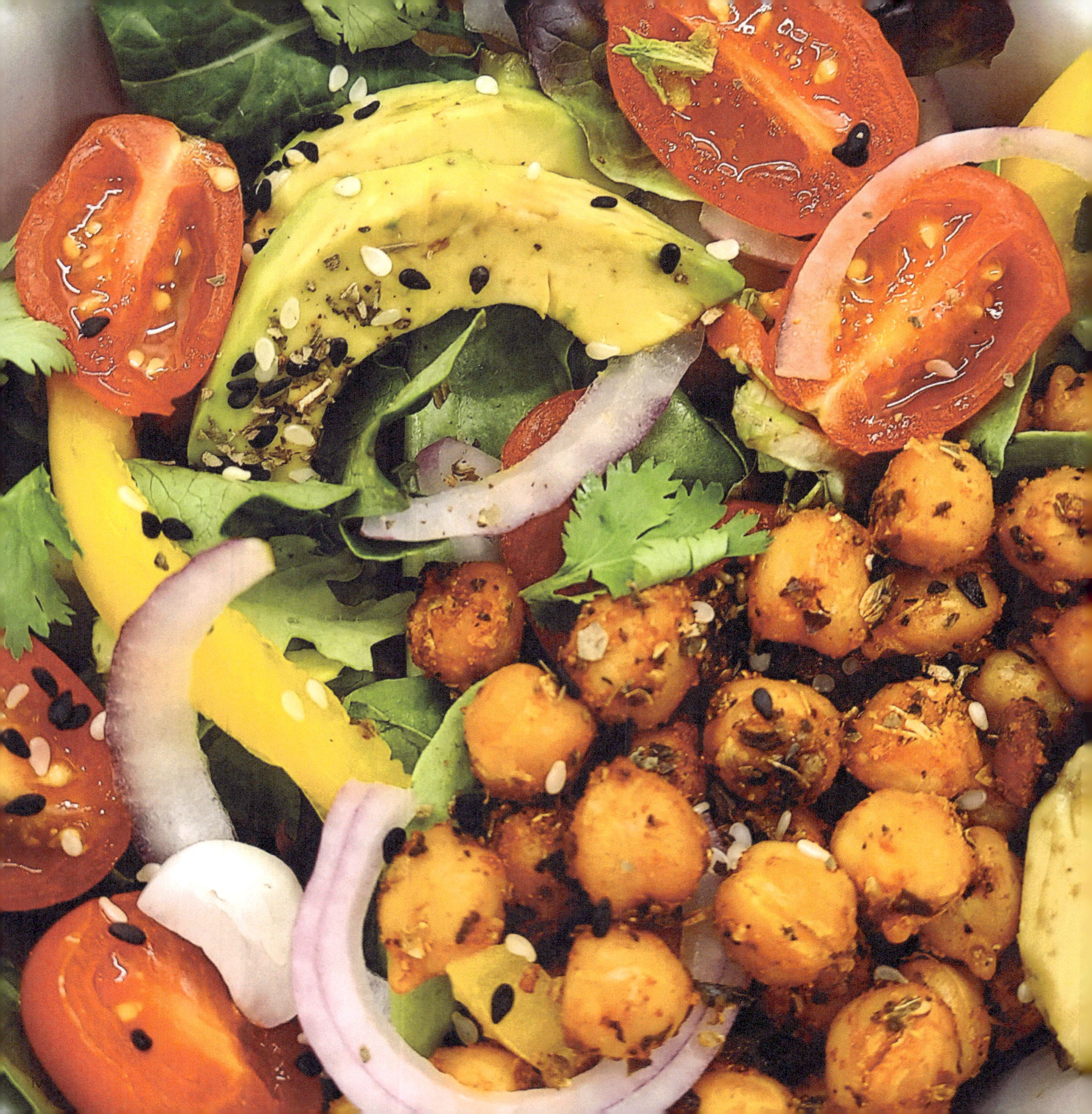

Organize Eating

A Cookbook for Transitioning to Plant-Based Meals

BEVERLY A. FLEMINGS

OTBE

For more information: Beverly@organizingtobeeffective.com

First paperback edition 2021
This book is not intended as a substitute for medical recommendation of physicians or other health-care providers. We advise readers to carefully review and understand the ideas presented and to seek advice of a qualified medial professional before you attempt to use them.

ISBN 978-0-578-68586-1 (paperback)
ISBN 978-0-9771388-2-1 (e-book)

Library of Congress Cataloging-in-Publication Data
Names: Flemings, Beverly A, Author
Title: Organize Eating: A Cookbook for Transitioning to Plant-Based Meals

Photographs by Beverly A. Flemings - (except Page 40, Herbs & spices (unsplash); page 217 Beverage- Dessert(unsplash)

Food Styling and Prop Styling by Beverly A. Flemings

Book Cover design by Michele Tate

This book is

**DEDICATED TO MY GRANDDAUGHTER,
KENNEDY NICOLE**

Who encouraged me to prepare her favorite dishes
and inspired me to write down the process.

TABLE OF CONTENTS

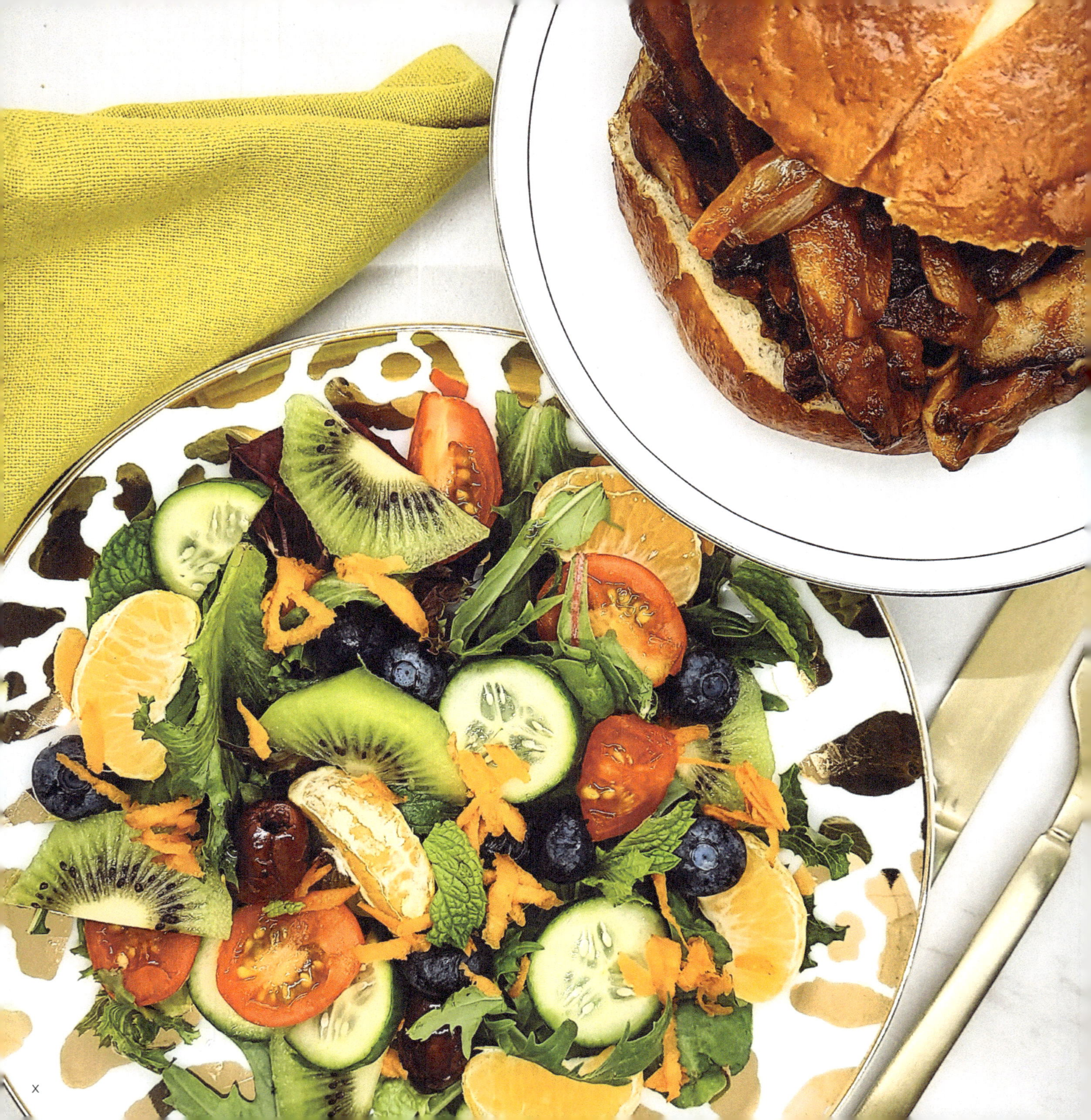

INTRODUCTION

What began over 35 years ago as a mere curiosity has become a call to action for my life. Food, in every form, growing it, shopping for it, preparing, enjoying eating and sharing it – I appreciate it all. My years of learning about food is a wonderful journey that evolved over time into the healthy lifestyle which has fared me well through raising two healthy children, a cancer diagnosis and general health as I age.

As I talk with people daily in markets and stores, at street vendors, in class and while working I find people from all walks of life are desiring change in their eating habits, lifestyle and health. Many people feel confused as to where to start. Even more people are unsure how to maintain their new health-wise eating without an organized process.

Today I understand and believe that one key to achieving and sustaining good health begins with our initial intention, then food selection and preparation. Learning to choose foods that increase your health and longevity comes from knowledge we gain on the subject. Wisdom, knowledge and understanding is needed to be healthy. Choose the highest quality of food you can afford. The quality of the ingredients will be reflected in the delicious dishes you prepare. Your food storage and preparation are vitally important to the life of the food you select. I know first hand that healthy food selection and preparation will promote and sustain a healthy body.

When I think of the simplest and least confusing method of transitioning from the Standard American Diet (SAD) to more plant based eating I reference what I did myself in the early 1970's. We know that change is a process – take the time to learn how your body functions and grow in the knowledge you learn daily. Embrace your new freedom to allow new habits to take shape and be inspired. You begin freeing yourself to truly learn how to live life more abundantly. I simply began going to a Farmer's Market (Eastern Market in Detroit, Michigan) every Saturday. I began to familiarize myself with the food. I purchased vegetables, talked with the farmers; and learned about their products. I returned home with the freshest food available in my area to prepare dishes for my family. All week I would work with the food I had chosen. Sometimes the food included vegetables I hadn't eaten as a child, many times vegetables I never heard of. My reference was basically the library in those days, other mothers and women and men who were more advanced in natural food selection and preparation than I. All of this happened before the explosion of the internet (at least for me) and the multitude of resources we now have at our disposal. I wasn't confused at all – very focused and very motivated. At dinner time I can remember my two little children would look at each other and then at their plates before taking their spoons and digging in - never knowing what mom had prepared. The children were not raised to say, "I don't like this" until they tried the food on their plates. Some foods were new to them and they liked; some they were not that enthused about, but they cleaned their plates regardless.

Not much has changed in my Saturday market routine; I do basically the same today as I did in the 70's. On Saturdays, March - December, I'm at the Market. I may visit multiple Farmers' Markets on Saturdays now, still talk to the farmers and others and return home with fresh, (mostly organic) vegetables for the week. The wonderful part is that now, unlike in the early 1970's during the winter months I can go to markets that specialize in the whole, organic, fresh foods I have grown to love. It is my hope that you enjoy and prosper in your food and health journey as much as I have. Writing this book has allowed me to share information, continue to learn and grow and to join with you on a amazing journey of health and wellness.

HOW TO USE THIS BOOK

This book is intended as a cooking aid and tool for transitioning into plant-based eating. If you are new to plant-based eating, there may be foods you have never prepared. The unfamiliar can be unnerving or unsettling, just know, that is true of being a "newbie" in any area.

Pointers to use the cookbook

1. It is best to read a recipe all the way through first. Some recipes require advance preparation, such as pre-cooking quinoa, pre-soaking dried beans, etc.
2. The cookbook represents seasonal cooking. Four sections in the book are organized around four seasons of the year – even though there are 6 seasons of food.
3. For people with medical challenges, the recipes are not a recommendation for healing. When I was diagnosed with a medical challenge, I followed a strict healing diet. I began adding foods back after being cleared and free of the challenge for a minimum of 2 years. Always check with your healthcare practitioner.
4. Sea salt is used in the recipes. If you are a no-salt user, simply do not add salt. Many people have good reason not to use salt. I use Light Grey Celtic sea salt, a mineral rich, whole crystal moist salt unrefined and hand harvested, in the recipes.
5. You will not find white sugar, white flour or white rice used in any recipes.
6. The farmer's market is a great resource for the plant-based diet. There are items

mentioned you may not find in a supermarket because the growing season is so short. For example, green garlic only lasts until the garlic is mature. Farmers may have it, but you won't find it in a supermarket. If you do not shop at farmer's market, no problem. This book is about transition.

7. Use the recipes as a template, only as you are confident to do so. Enjoy good food and good health.

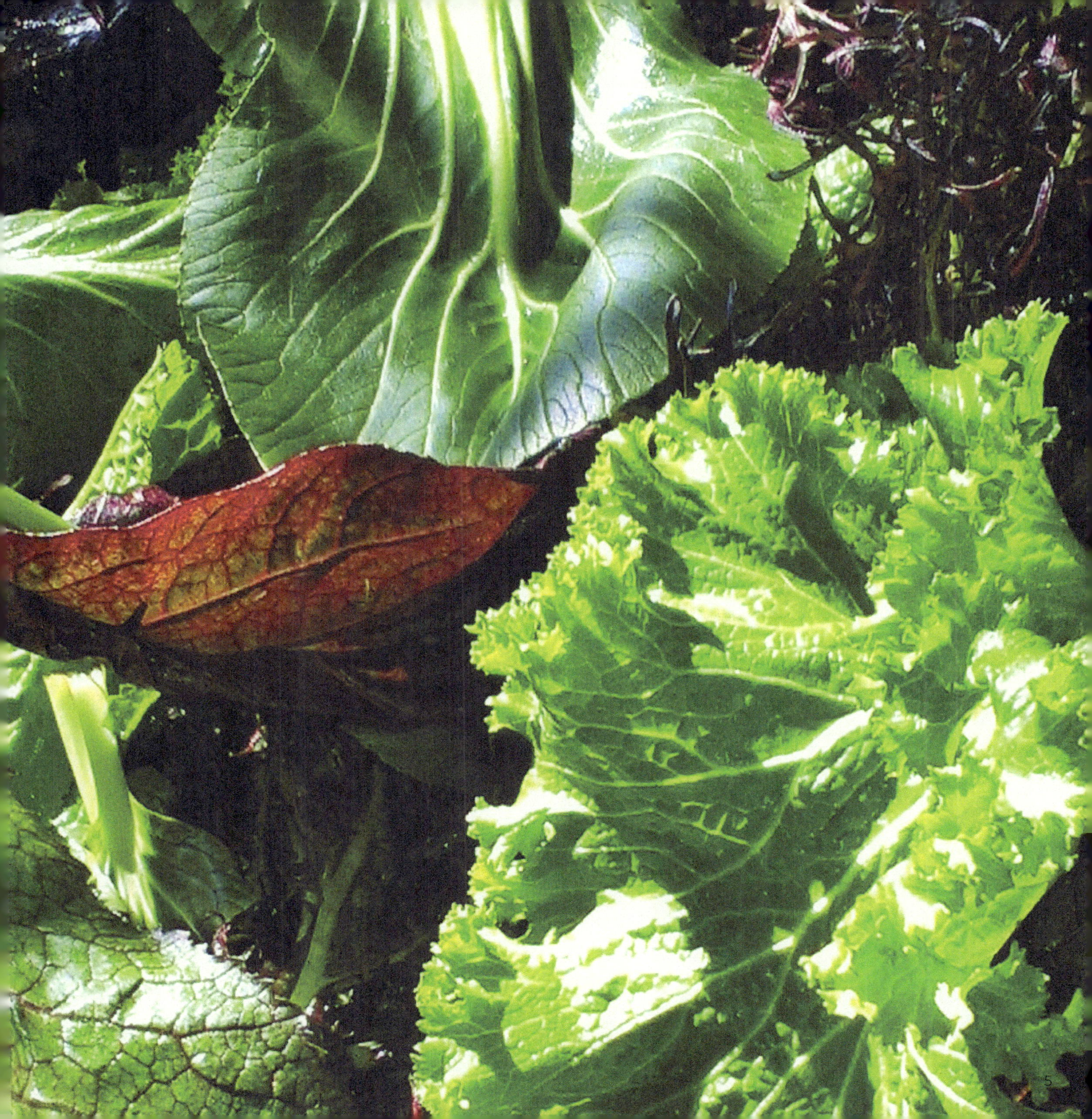

To every thing there is a season,
and a time to every purpose
under the heaven:

Ecclesiastes 3:1

Seasonal Eating

Part One

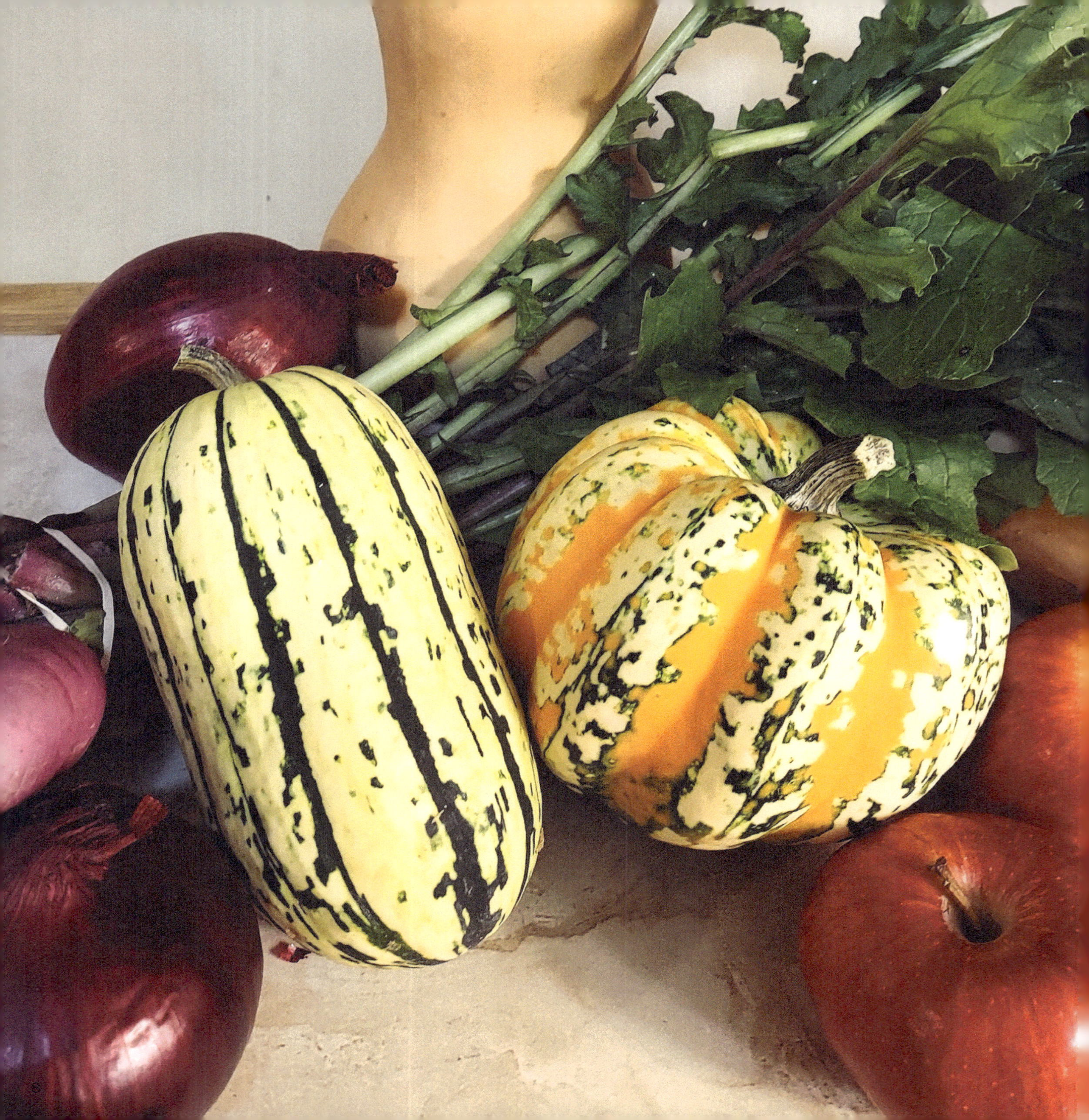

CHAPTER ONE

INTRODUCTION TO SEASONAL EATING

As you become more food-conscious, you will also become more aware of seasonal eating, a way of eating that gives you produce that is nutrient-rich and more cost effective. This is the way many people globally have eaten their whole lives. The heart of seasonal eating is gaining an understanding of the benefits of organizing meals around food that is currently in season and grown in your local community. There is a gentle unfolding of the seasons of the year (especially in Michigan). The seasons of life unfold in much the same way, naturally. It is to our health to flow with nature as much as possible.

The seasonality of food refers to the time of year when a given food type is at its peak, either in terms of its harvest (i.e., availability in markets) or its flavor. Those two factors usually coincide. How could you even compare a tomato picked locally in July to one picked unripe in December and then transported across the country? There is no comparison. The taste and flavor, the higher nutritional value, and the lower cost of the in-season tomato speak for themselves. Each year, I eagerly await locally grown tomatoes in the summer and apple cider in the fall. Being a foodie, I love anticipating the seasonal flavor of food when it's freshly harvested.

I have grown to appreciate seasonality so much, in fact, that I stopped eating tomatoes during the off-season months and replaced them with other foods. It took time to make that adjustment to a seasonal alternative. Now I experiment with and enjoy other produce in the fall, fruits and vegetables that I had never even considered putting on my salads before. Variety is the spice of life! I once asked my farmer why aren't asparagus harvested in November. In answer, he pointed up to the sky, meaning "God is in charge." Certain foods are grown in certain seasons, and as an organic farmer, he was growing food as God intended. I very much appreciate aligning with nature as much as possible.

The world over people go to the market daily to purchase local ingredients they use to prepare nutrient-rich, unprocessed meals. In many countries, this is all people know. Produce eaten at its peak generally has more antioxidants, vitamins, and minerals than produce shipped from distant locations. Shopping for fresh produce at local markets is also the way our grandparents ate, while our great-grandparents probably grew their produce.

SEASONAL

Seasonal eating means enjoying a variety of foods. As the seasons rotate so will the food we choose. Eating a variety of healthy, seasonal foods is an optimal way to receive a larger spectrum of vitamins and minerals that the body may be lacking. It's also an integral part of enjoying good health and emotional balance.

Too often, we stick with our favorite foods' year in and year out—it is so easy to indulge in the same dishes over and over again! Unfortunately, many of your favorite dishes may have very little (if any) nutritional value but have become a quick go-to family favorite out of convenience. It's wise to be open-minded and to learn about the benefits of eating a rainbow of foods. Not only is eating seasonal, a cost-effective way to eat, you will gain firsthand knowledge and experience of the flavors, tastes, and textures of a wider assortment of foods. Seasonal eating is simple, healthy, and good for the environment.

"To every thing, there is a season..." (Ecclesiastes 3:1). Within the seasons, nature really does have it all figured out! In the spring, we can start our inner cleansing with bitter, detoxifying greens such as dandelion leaf, kale, and parsley. Summer brings an abundance of hydrating fruits and vegetables, like cucumbers, tomatoes, watermelons, and summer squash that cool our bodies—hydration through fruit provides the natural water source our system needs. In the fall, we are greeted with apples, pears, pomegranates, cranberries, mushrooms, and squash...all delicious seasonal foods. (Apples are also good for detoxing as we begin to transition to cool temperatures.) In the winter, wonderful root vegetables give us the robust nutrition we need as temperatures drop. As year-end arrives, we transition to slow-cooking foods and drinking more warming liquids and teas. Herbs like sage, rosemary, and thyme are healing for the body and add vigor to winter dishes. Spices like cinnamon and ginger gently warm us and increase circulation.

Learning to keep our bodies in sync with nature is a secret to a healthy and extended life. Seasonal eating also embodies a sense of family and community. So which foods should you enjoy each season to increase your well-being? Well, the average person may not be familiar with complex nutritional facts, but the simple choice to eat seasonally is very basic and uncomplicated. Plus, with your choice, you support the local economy, community, and local/urban farmers.

LOCAL

Without a doubt, the freshest foods available to you are from your own garden or from local farmers in your area. Local farmers generally sell food as it becomes available—it's often picked the previous day or even that morning. It doesn't get much better than that! There are numerous ways you can interact with local farmers: local farms, farmer's markets, CSAs, farm stands, u-pick produce, etc. Over time, you will develop bonds and build relationships with your farmers. Look for these opportunities in your area:

- Community-supported agriculture (CSA) has become a popular way for consumers to buy local, seasonal food directly from a farmer. Here are the basics: a farmer offers a certain number of "shares" to the public, and interested consumers purchase a share (a.k.a. a "membership" or a "subscription"). In return, members receive a box/bag/basket of seasonal produce each week throughout the farming season. Typically, the share consists of a box of vegetables, but other farm products may be included. For more information, see: https://www.localharvest.org/csa/

- Farmer's markets: Spring signals the return of farmer's markets! When it comes to learning about food, meeting farmers, and purchasing farm-fresh food nothing compares to the farmer's market. Besides freshly picked vegetables, many markets also offer seasonal fruits, grains, legumes, sprouts, eggs, and garlic, to name a few items. You may also find local honey and maple syrup along and an opportunity to support the farming community!

ORGANIC

The word "organic" refers to the way farmers grow and process agricultural products, such fruits, vegetables, grains, dairy products, and meat. Organic farming practices are designed to reduce pollution and encourage soil and water conservation—farmers who grow organic produce and meat don't use conventional methods to fertilize, control weeds, or prevent livestock disease. For example, organic farmers may conduct crop rotations and spread mulch or manure to keep weeds at bay rather than using chemical weed killers. The U.S. Department of Agriculture (USDA) has established an organic certification program that requires all organic foods to meet strict government standards that regulate how such foods are grown, handled, and processed.

Products certified 95 percent or more organic can display the USDA sticker. If a food bears a USDA organic label, that means it was produced and processed according to USDA standards and that at least 95 percent of the food's ingredients were organically produced. The seal is voluntary, but many organic producers use it.

Single-ingredient products (fruits, vegetables, etc.) that are completely organic are labeled as being 100 percent organic and can carry a USDA seal. Foods that have more than one ingredient (breakfast cereals, breads, etc.) can use the USDA organic seal or the following wording on their package labels, depending on the number of organic ingredients:

- "100 percent organic." Products that are completely made of organic ingredients.
- "Organic." Products that are at least 95 percent organic.
- "Made with organic ingredients." These products contain at least 70 percent organic ingredients. The organic seal can't be used on these products.
- Foods containing less than 70 percent organic ingredients can't use the organic seal on their product label, but they can include the organic items in their ingredient list: for example, "organic apples" rather than "apples" if they are in fact organic.

You may see other terms on food labels, such as "all-natural," "free-range," or" hormone-free." These descriptions may be important to you, but don't confuse them with the term "organic." Only those foods that are grown and processed according to USDA organic standards can be labeled organic.

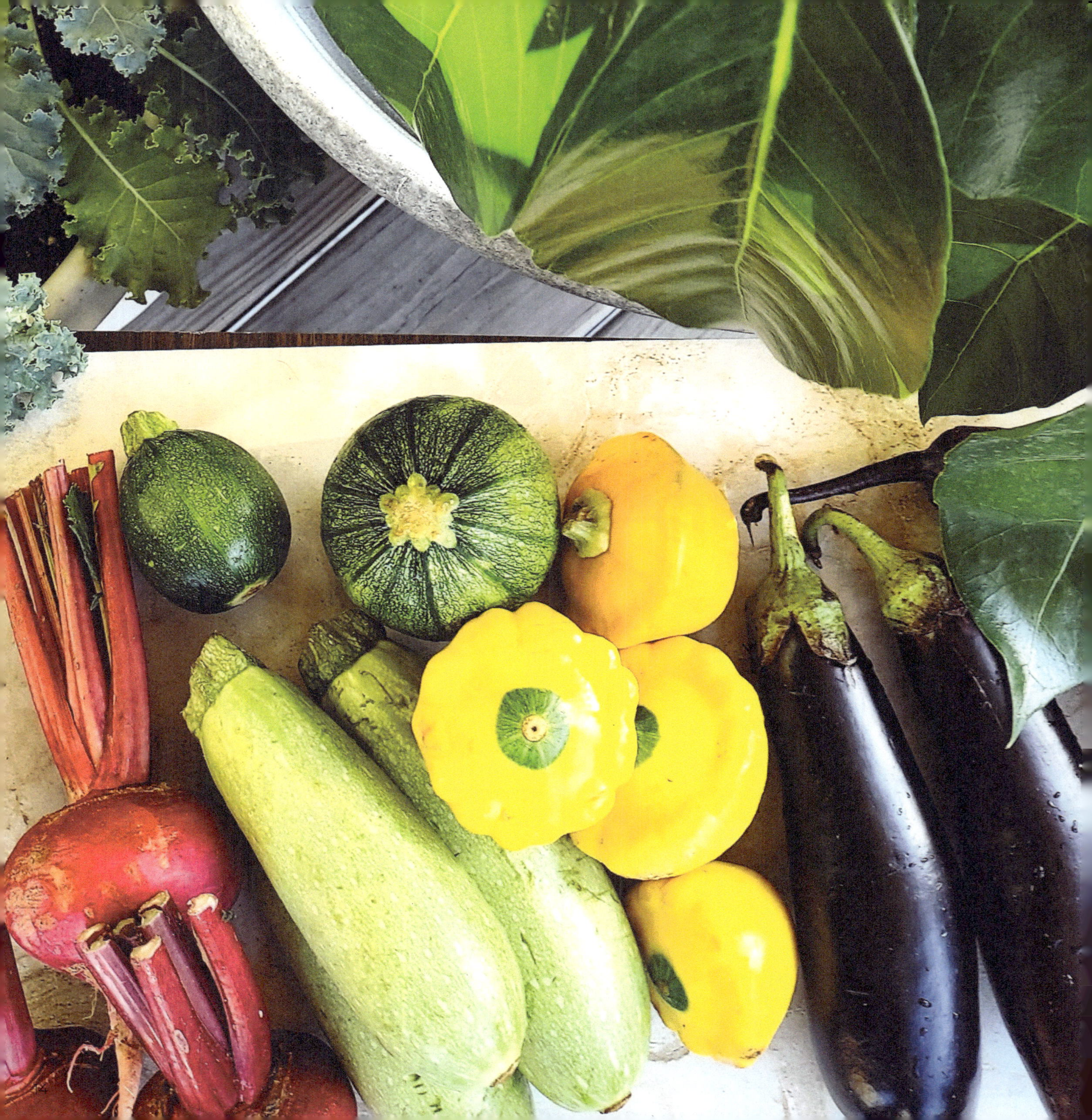

CHAPTER TWO

ORGANIZING FOR A NEW LIFESTYLE

A healthy eating lifestyle is very much about what is in your kitchen. In short that means; your food choices, food storage, food preparation can represent a brand-new lifestyle. Meal planning is not only about planning, it is also about implementing. With thoughtful meal planning, it is easy to get pumped up about the healthy meals you plan to prepare throughout the week! It is even easier to get busy and sometimes fall short of your goal because of a lack of organization.

Putting plans into action does take coordination, but not a lot. Meal planning is built around thinking ahead and preparing. Having order in your life will help move your new lifestyle forward. The term "lifestyle" is being used more frequently. It's called "lifestyle" because the style of your life changes. More specifically the way you choose to live your life is changing as you move or transition into a new way of thinking. Changes can include selecting food differently, read labels before purchasing, and be more mindful of what you eat. These are changes in your style of living not merely changes in your eating.

Lifestyle embodies your attitude, the way you view the world, and what you want for yourself. Your life is taking on a new style, as you acquire new habits. Introducing new thoughts, habits and routines are lifestyle changes. Embrace that new style because it is moving you forward and forward movement only happens when we are ready!

As a professional organizer I've chosen (or maybe it chose me) to introduce order as a tool for effectiveness. Being effective is different from being efficient. Becoming better organized, or more effective, is a process that can make a healthy lifestyle so much easier! The principles of organize eating thrive in a healthy, safe kitchen where you can enjoy the pleasure of preparing nutritious, delicious meals. Organizing is a tool to assist you. Let's talk about it.

An organized, healthy kitchen can become a center of wholeness for you, your family, and even your community. A clean kitchen floor, stovetop, oven, counter, pantry and a fresh-smelling refrigerator are all part of your new healthy lifestyle. Your physical kitchen is as important to your health goals as a pot of quinoa or a morning smoothie. Make your kitchen become a comfortable environment that supports your mental and physical well-being. Organizing is a powerful tool to help you achieve that. Organizing is a very freeing process that makes your life better! Establishing order in your home can relieve the stress and frustration that would otherwise steal your joy.

The organizing process begins with a mindset of establishing order. "Order" has a different meaning for each person, of course, but the desire and need for order begins in the mind and can ultimately transform your entire life. This happens because organizing is an intentional activity. If you are not intentional in your pursuit of adding order, there is a great possibility it, won't happen for you. Many times people settle for neatness, which is an example of efficiency, whether than organization, which is an example of effectiveness. Here is the good news: you do not need to be an organizing superstar. You do not need to understand all the fundamentals of the organizing process to be better organized. You do, however, need to make clarity, structure, and consistency priorities in your life in order to be transformed by the process of organizing.

Having a clutter-free, peaceful home is a gift. As you honor your living space with order, you create a sanctuary, the supportive environment we each need. You invite health, wholeness, and prosperity to thrive in your life and in your home.

"I wish above all things that you prosper and be in health even as your soul prospers." (3 John 1:2)

Let's be honest—your mind, your will, and your emotions cannot prosper amid clutter and confusion.

Many people are re-discovering their creativity in the kitchen and their love of home cooking. If you don't feel that way yet, remember that it just takes a little planning to take away the fear of the unknown. Committing to a healthier lifestyle does not have to be a daunting task! I've written ***Organize Eating: A Cookbook for Transitioning into Plant-Based Meals*** to help you to move forward, one step at a time. I personally endorse one step at a time transition. Many things about your life will change. Relax and allow the changes to unfold naturally without you rushing the process to duplicate what you may view on social media. Each life journey is unique. Live your own story of health and wholeness. Learn about your body and how to be healthy for real inside and outside.

While there are wonderful vegan, plant-based and vegetarian food restaurants, it may be difficult to change your eating lifestyle if you are continuously eating out. At some point, you might want to cook at home. As you begin to appreciate wholesome food, preparing healthy meals will be a great inspiration for you. There is no way around it—as the saying goes, "We are what we eat." Eating a nutritious diet can give you a sense of harmony and well-being, improve your health, slow the aging process, and help you maintain a balanced weight. I believe the more knowledgeable you become the more in control and less fearful you will be. Knowledge is power!

KITCHEN ESSENTIALS

Kitchen essentials are utensils, appliances, and equipment you use in your home kitchen. These tools also reinforce your cooking style. My first kitchen tools were: a knife, a pot, a pan and a cast-iron skillet. I was so excited when I finally added my juice extractor. I still have that Champion juicer—the motor can grind up a tree trunk! Today there are an ever-increasing variety of kitchen gadgets and tools in stores. The new, innovative kitchen appliances save time in the kitchen, improve how recipes are prepared, and give home cooking a modern makeover. The right equipment can take the guesswork out of cooking!

Below are the kitchen tools used to prepare the recipes in this book. I did not begin cooking with most of these but through the years have come to rely on them. Start where you are - add as you can.

- Anti-fatigue mat –non-slip top -bottom surface provides, comfort, safety and relief
- Baking pan/rimmed baking sheet – a metal pan with raised sides used in the oven
- Baking sheet (flat) – a metal pan with no raised sides used in the oven
- Blender – electric appliance used for blending/mixing food
- Bowls – assorted sizes used for mixing, storage and serving
- Box grater – tool used for hand grating
- Citrus juicer – tool used to juice citrus fruit
- Colander – a bowl-shaped utensil used to drain food
- Cutting boards (wooden is best) – durable boards used for cutting and chopping
- Knives – chef knife (multi- purpose knife), paring knife (peeling), Santoku knife
- Juice extractor – to extract juice from fruit, leafy greens and other types of vegetables
- Measuring cups/spoons – to measure an amount in standard measurement sizes
- Mini chopper – a small electric appliance for chopping small amounts
- Nutri-bullet – nutrient extractor: makes veggie and fruit based drinks and soups
- Parchment paper – used when baking to create a clean, non-stick surface

- Pots - different sizes; larger pot has two handles usually used for cooking liquid
- Salad spinner – to wash/remove excess water from greens
- Sauté pan – flat-bottomed pan with long handle for cooking on top of the stove
- Skillets (cast-iron and stainless steel) – pans for cooking on top of the stove or in oven
- Strainers – perforated metal sieve for straining food (pasta, rice, grains, etc.)
- Utensils (wooden) – wooden utensils don't scratch the surface of pots/pans
- Vegetable peeler – prepping tool for peeling vegetable

ORDER IN THE KITCHEN

When it comes to organizing the kitchen, here's how to start:

- Make a Quality Decision
- Set Aside Time
- Create a Plan
- Stay on Point

The amount of time you spend getting things in order is not as important as your being consistent. Commit to and work at adding order consistently, even if you just spend 15 to 30 minutes a day getting things organized. The key is to stay purposeful and committed. When you do, the process will give your mind a new focus point. Allow that focus point to draw you along with the flow of it.

You already have the kitchen, your focus is to bring your existing environment into alignment with your vision of a new lifestyle. Having an environment that supports your new lifestyle is an investment and a joy. **An organized kitchen will bring you satisfaction every day as you continue to invest in your health! The joy you will experience has very little to do with the size of your kitchen or the number of appliances you own—instead, it has everything to do with your attitude and the goals you set towards health, food, and food preparation. Begin where you are, and awesome meals will follow.**

One of the best ways to ensure success as you move into healthier eating choices is to create a kitchen you enjoy being and cooking in. As you intentionally make lifestyle changes, various details will begin to move in the direction of your intentions. The kitchen is multi-functional, no matter the size. It is a place where you will handle many tasks and will use numerous appliances and pieces of equipment for food preparation. You can begin to establish order anywhere you fancy. Organizing your kitchen need not happen in one day! Take time and think about the what, where, when, and how of your specific kitchen. Organizing a kitchen is mainly about functionality—form follows function. That simply means how the space functions for you is more important than its décor. Your household needs will also dictate how you want to organize your kitchen. There may be a lot going on in your kitchen! Always remember the kitchen has a specific role to perform because it is the center of family life. A center for health and wholeness.

Whether you are in an apartment, condo, or house, the kitchen is where people love to gather, mainly because of the food, the smells of food, the warmth of the kitchen, and good ol' hospitality. Many modern kitchens have enlarged layouts and are very accommodating places for people to gather. Even in tiny kitchens, people come into the kitchen for nourishment. They ask, "What's cooking?" Whatever is in the pot can make a difference in the well-being of family and friends. You have the power right there in that space to share a healthy variety of food with people who trust your judgment. A growing number of people are moving into healthier eating habits, and many are considering plant-based meals. This is generating a real shift in home cooking. What a great time to return to the kitchen!

Just think—by adding a little order, you'll be able to open your refrigerator and clearly see what you have on hand. With clear counter space and your ingredients within hand's reach, it is easier to chop, dice, and be creative with ingredients. This is true whether your kitchen is large or small. Being organized eliminates clutter and establishes order. Clutter comes in many forms, and unfortunately, all forms of clutter are destructive.

As you continue establishing a new order, your kitchen will soon become a center of wellness and health, a place of nourishment for you and those you care about. Since the kitchen is referred to as the heart of the home, our personal habits and established routines are what make a health-orientated HOME. The best meals are prepared where harmony flows. Order and harmony will help you be more creative when planning meals and will enable you to enjoy the kitchen! It can also provide you with time to think and work with a calm assurance that the dishes you prepare will be delicious and nutritious.

The questions below can help you better allocate space in your kitchen, pantry, and refrigerator.

ORGANIZING SURVEY FOR YOUR KITCHEN SETUP

1. Are you organizing as a:

   ◻ single person ◻ family (how many? __) or ◻ community?

2. How many cooks are in the kitchen? _____ Do you need a child-friendly kitchen?

   ____

   ____

   ____

3. What is the predominant eating style? ____________________

   ____

   ____

4. How much space is needed for kitchen equipment? ____________________

   ____

   ____

5. Is food being prepared to be eaten at: ☐ home, ☐ work, or ☐ school? ____________

6. How often do you grocery shop? ________ Is food purchased in quantities? _______
____
____

7. Is the kitchen used for other home activities? ______________________________
____
____

Notes:
____
____

FOOD SELECTION

Selecting food with care is where we start. As your eating habits transition, so will your food selection.

The joy of a healthy lifestyle comes with the personal responsibility to identify and select the foods for optimal health. Choosing foods that are safe, nourish your body, provide the energy and healing properties needed to maintain good health is the goal.

The main thought here is, the food you bring into your homes, store in your pantry and refrigerator is what you have on hand to prepare meals, and reach for when you are hungry. No one comes into this world with a desire for any of the foods you wind up eating as an adult. It is all learned behavior. You have learned to eat the way you do, and you are able to change that narrative when you choose. Choose foods that lead to health and life.

Our meals come from a variety of places which include: meals made from scratch, carry out meals brought home, meals made at home with pre-prepared frozen or packaged food and the list goes on. Regardless of the food source, many foods are packaged for preservation. The food is packaged in cans, bottles, jars and packages using numerous methods to prevent food from spoilage and to extend the shelf life of the food. It is important to read labels and become aware of the ingredients (i.e., possible hazards) used in the preservation of these foods. It is wise to understand what is in the packaged foods you consume.

This checklist can help organize your plant-based food selection:

1. Understanding Food Labels - know what you are eating
2. Inventory what you have on hand and write a list before shopping
3. Select a variety of foods—learn to eat a rainbow
4. Select food using your senses.
5. Select the highest quality of food you can afford. Let's re-define wha a bargain is.

UNDERSTANDING FOOD LABELS

Food labeling is important. Labels help you understand the composition of your food: its vitamins, minerals, calories, fats, and more. This information is fundamental in ensuring that you are eating the kinds of food that are good for you. "The Food and Drug Administration (FDA) is responsible for assuring that foods sold in the United States are safe, wholesome and properly labeled. This applies to foods produced domestically, as well as foods from foreign countries. The Nutrition Labeling and Education Act (NLEA), which amended the FD&C Act, requires most foods to bear nutrition labeling and requires food labels that bear nutrient content claims and certain health messages to comply with specific requirements."

When looking at the Nutrition Facts label, first take a look at the serving information.

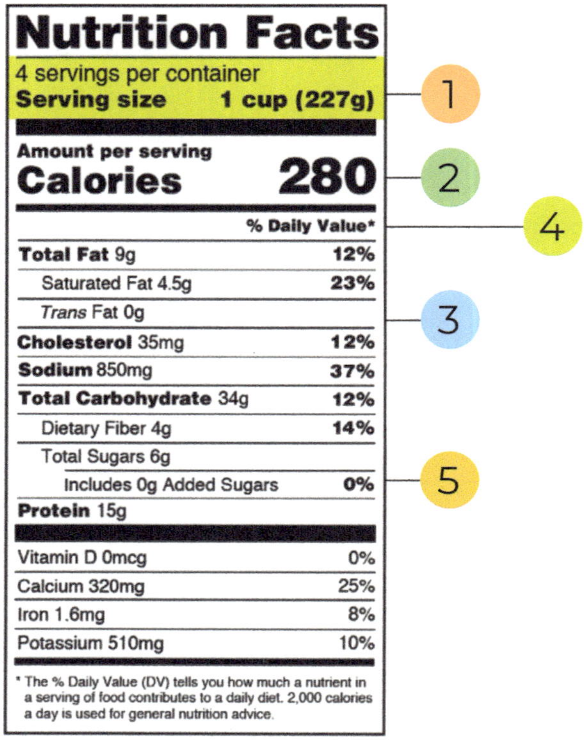

Serving Information (1): This includes the number of servings in the package (servings per container) and the serving size. Serving sizes are standardized to make it easier to compare similar foods; they are provided in familiar units, such as cups or pieces, followed by the metric amount, e.g., the number of grams (g).

The serving size is not a recommendation of how much you should eat or drink. It's important to realize that all the nutrient amounts shown on the label, including the number of calories, are dependent on the serving size.

Pay attention to the serving size, especially how many servings there are in the food package. For example, you might ask yourself if you are consuming ½ serving, 1 serving, or more. In the sample label, one serving of soup equals 1 cup. If you ate two cups, you would be consuming two servings. That is two times the nutrients shown in the sample label, so you would need to double the these amounts, as well as the %DVs, to know what you are getting in two servings. For example, if you ate 2 cups of this soup, you would be eating 560 calories.

Calories (2): For most consumers, calories are often considered before anything else. However, calories can be obtained from healthy or unhealthy options. Real, wholefoods are comprised of so many components beyond calories. They are packed with fiber, vitamins, minerals, and phytonutrients such as antioxidants. For example, these options have about the same number of calories: A can of Coca-Cola (140 calories), one tablespoon of cooking oil (120 calories), one large apple (116 calories), or four cups of broccoli (124 calories). Although they are similar in calories, their overall nutrition varies greatly. The point: Look beyond calories.

Nutrients (3): The food label lists some nutrients such as fat, protein, carbohydrates, fiber, and some vitamins and minerals. Some nutrients we want to be high, such as fiber, whereas others are best to keep low, such as added sugars. The food label provides a quick snapshot of our essential nutrients, yet does not list all of the vitamins and minerals and it does not list phytonutrients, discussed more in the following section.
The point: Eat a wide range of colorful, whole foods and you will benefit from the nutrients listed on the food label and much more!

Percent daily value (%DV) (4): %DV can help determine if there is a high or low amount of a nutrient in a food. If %DV is 5% or lower, the food is low in that nutrient. If %DV is 20% or higher, the food is high in that nutrient. For example, the above food label shows that one cup of the soup contains about 37% DV of sodium, so this is a high-sodium food. Again, keep in mind the serving size. If you ate 2 cups of the food, this is twice as much sodium, which is 74% DV of sodium!

Added Sugars (5): Just below Total Sugars, you will see Added Sugars listed on the food label. This tells us which sugars are processed and have been added to the food product, such as high fructose corn syrup or sucrose (white table sugar). Added sugars are different than naturally-occurring sugars, which can be found in real, whole foods such as fruits or starchy vegetables. Total sugars is the total of the added sugars and the naturally-occurring sugars. Looking at the example, one cup of soup has 6g of total sugars, yet 0g of added sugars. This tells us that the soup contains 6g of naturally-occurring sugars, since it does not contain any added sugars. The American Heart Association recommends less than 24g of added sugars daily for women and less than 36g of added sugars for men. To visualize this in teaspoons, the limit for women is 6 teaspoons daily and the limit for men is 9 teaspoons daily. Keep in mind this is a maximum recommendation and our bodies do not require added sugars in any amount to function well. Instead, naturally-occurring sugars from whole, plant foods provide optimal energy.

FOOD SELECTION

The joy of a healthy lifestyle comes with a personal responsibility to identify and select the foods for optimal health. Choosing foods that are safe, nourish your body, provide the energy and healing properties needed to maintain good health is the goal.

This checklist can help organize your plant-based food selection:

☐ **Inventory Before Shopping –**

Surveying what you have on hand can make it easy to:

- Know what foods you have at home
- Create a grocery list of items you want to return home with
    - Use paper or a digital device (cell phone, iPad)
- Stay on healthy eating plan – by committing to the grocery list
- Save time - grocery shopping
- Save money by purchasing from your list

☐ **Select A Variety Of Foods – Eat A Rainbow**

- Eating a variety of colorful foods will give you a full range of vitamins and mineral the body needs to thrive.
- The colorful pigments in fruits and vegetables are produced by specific phytonutrients, which are natural chemicals produced in plants.
- These pigments represent various micronutrients that are essential for good health.
- Each color indicates an abundance of specific nutrients that the body needs.
- Pigments may change due to an alkaline or acid condition or certain reactive metals.

Some natural food pigments:

- Orange - yellow foods: Beta-Carotene - immune system and eye help
- Green foods: Chlorophyll - blood and bone health
- Blue – purple – red: Anthocyanins - anti-cancer, anti-aging

- Red foods - help fight cancer, heart disease
- White and brown: certain cancers, bones and heart

☐ **Selecting Produce By Your Senses** – Makes good sense!
We learn **to use** our senses when selecting produce along with personal experience and data.

Our eyes: to view the freshness of foods. Wilted, discolored leaves are not fresh. Bruised, shriveled, or damaged items are not to be chosen.

- Broccoli: yellow florets not chosen
- Celery: should be green not lime (the darker the better)
- Eggplant: shiny, firm, unblemished
- Leafy greens: collards, kale, should be dark green, no yellow, water saturated leaves
- Pomegranate: unblemished; firm with a little give

Our hands: feel the weight, firmness, also the texture of a food.

- Asparagus: avoid limp stalk
- Avocados: a little give is best, not too soft and not too hard.
- Green Bean: snap them, limp not chosen
- Onions: shiny skin is best, no soft spots or sprouts growing
- Root vegetables: no cracks at the base, no wrinkled skin

Our nose: smelling food is helpful in identifying fresh versus spoiled foods. Especially in the summer, the fragrance of fruit and vegetables alike is an indicator of freshness.

- Fruit: fresh vs. spoiling (learn the smell + view the fruit)
- Onions: pungent smell;
- Pineapple: light sweet smell; yellow color from bottom up
- Melons: light sweet smell; watch out for strong smell and too soft touch
- Tomatoes: earthy smell; firm but not hard; not too soft

☐ Select The Highest Quality Food You Can Afford

We hear the saying "we are what we eat." more frequently. For the food we eat to nourish at the cellular level (almost all food including fast food will reach the cellular level but not all foods will nourish at the cellular level), we have to eat food that is a high quality. PERIOD. Garage in is garbage out.

I believe that the highest quality of food is the food purchased from local farmers, either face-to-face at farmer's markets or through Community Supported Agriculture (CSA) boxes of produce that are sourced from the local farming community or food co-opt.You can also be your own farmer and produce your own high-quality produce! Quality products can typically be found in produce markets and stores plus we can also select food from markets if we are mindful and read labels. It's best to explore your own food community to learn where to go for what you need.

That being said, plant – based grocery days are how you grow to learn your personal terrain: where to go for the foods that you want. It is also how we build relationships with food providers. Talking to merchants, vendors, farmers, super market produce managers: this is true networking. I grew up at a time that Saturday was grocery shopping day. There was something in the air. People were in the streets with their shopping bags under their arms, many awaiting public transportation to go to the market, whether in the neighborhood or the Eastern Market and Grand Central Market. I learned to utilize these resources. For years. I joined in and learned the meaning of community. Talking to produce managers in super markets was a source I used long before the food scene became as populated with the variety of food it has now. If you were shopping for something special the merchant would show it to you and get your approval before wrapping up your selection. People took the time to shop for the best food they could afford. Then the spices, bay leaves, etc. would bring out the flavors. We are getting back to that type of food selection. The kind of shopping and gathering food leads to having a healthy body. We are also returning to healthy attitudes about our personal responsibility for our health and well-being.

FOOD SELECTION: There is more to whole food plant-based eating than fruit and vegetables. The following ingredients combined with the fruit and vegetables can make a rich, nutritious diet:

- Herbs: fresh and dried, add flavor, aroma, nutrients and texture to meals
- Spices: add flavor, aroma, nutrients and texture to food. Select whole or grounded
- Legumes: beans, peas, lentils – organic is best; locally grown if possible or canned
- Nuts and seeds: protein, healthy fats, vitamins, and minerals. Fresh as possible
- Sea vegetation: edible seaweed is a sea vegetable that absorbs iodine from the ocean
- Whole grain: unprocessed grain contains all original parts - the bran, germ and endosperm
  - "Look for the word "whole" in the first ingredient of a grain product to determine is whole grain. The words "enriched" or "refined" grains are not whole grain products."
- Soy products: from the soybean (an Asian legume) used to produce a number of products; used as a meat replacement (for vegetarians and vegans alike).
- Mushrooms: are classified as fungi, most mushrooms are a good source of selenium and potassium

FOOD STORAGE

Taking the time and responsibility to store food properly is a single act that will:

- Save you money
- Cut waste
- Keep you healthy

Where to start with food storage? The best place to start is where you are! I am a professional organizer, so my forte is order, not neatness ORDER. Food storage isn't as much about being neat and efficient, as it is about being organized and effective. It is about accessibility. We will eat what is in our homes and within easy reach. Like proper food selection, proper food storage is setting you up to live a healthier life, not about having food neatly positioned on a shelf.

Order is how you think and what you think about, and in this case, the thought is to be in health and to be free of sickness, disease or pain. This is the order that organization comes from. Organizing your thoughts and thinking through your life choices.

Let's look at two storage units in the kitchen that will keep us on track with healthier eating: the pantry and the refrigerator.

A WELL-STOCKED PANTRY

A well-stocked pantry is the essence to successful home cooking. Your pantry can give you peace of mind. Why is that, you may ask? Because a well-stocked pantry is a collection of the basic ingredients you have chosen, ingredients you want and need to prepare delicious, nutritious meals. A well-stocked pantry does not mean overstocked—it means your pantry is stocked with a selection of your go-to ingredients for creating healthy meals. Your new lifestyle change starts with your pantry, so take time to be choosy about the pantry foods you purchase. When you use a new ingredient and are pleased with the results, make that item a staple. (Tip: don't overstock your pantry with items just because they may be on sale.)

As a general rule, cluttered, overstocked, disorganized cupboards and pantries are often full of unhealthy food choices. A well-stocked pantry, on the other hand, contains a selective variety of ingredients that allows you to be creative, health-conscious, inspired and even adventurous when you want to whip something up. Cooking is how you will learn how uncomplicated it is to prepare healthy and delicious dishes and meals. It's worth taking time to write out your pantry list (itemized by categories), because then you also have a handy grocery list. You may want to post the list close to the pantry and check to see which items you need to replace and which new items you'll need to look for when you go shopping. If you are a digital or high tech person, there is a wide variety of food shopping and meal planning apps. Carrying your shopping list electronically is handy. Remember the Milk is a wonderful app for busy people.

Creating a pantry list allows you to:

- Know what you have on hand
- Save time and money when shopping
- Develop an organized way of planning ahead
- Quickly organize wholesome meals, snacks and appetizers

Food staples are regularly used perishable and non-perishable items that a cook selects to keep on hand.

Perishable staple foods are foods to use before they spoil. Examples of these include:

- Carrots
- Celery
- Onions
- Garlic

Nonperishable staples are dry goods that keep for an extended time in storage. Examples of these include:

- Dry beans
- Whole grains
- Flour
- Dry seasonings

As you continue to organize and cultivate your pantry, your kitchen will soon become a center of wellness and health. Since the kitchen is often referred to as the heart of the home, our personal habits and established routine make it HOME. Establishing order in the kitchen is what will make the kitchen an inviting space. Order can help you be creative and have fun! Order can also provide you with the time to think and work with a calm assurance that the dishes you prepare will be delicious and nutritious. Clutter, on the other hand, will disrupt the flow from food prep to cooking each time you have to stop to clear off more counter space or search for ingredients.

A well-stocked pantry eliminates the need to go grocery shopping every time you prepare a meal. Whether your pantry is a cupboard cabinet, shelves of containers over your sink or a custom-built walk-in doesn't matter. What does matter is that you fill your pantry with ingredients that inspire you and assist you in creating hearty, healthy dishes. The physical pantry is simply a vehicle of convenience, an organizing tool that allows you to be effective in your kitchen. Cooking is not a one-size-fits-all endeavor, so there's no such thing as a one-size-fits-all pantry. Your cooking and eating style is reflected in the ingredients you keep on hand in your pantry, cupboards and refrigerator.

There is no need to stock your pantry all at once—simply purchase or gather the items you use often, ingredients you want to have on hand. (By "gathering," I am referring to items you make or items your neighbors and friends give you, such as preserves, jams, jars of cha-cha, etc.). Build up your pantry gradually. Perishables such as fresh fruits and vegetables are not considered pantry items—these items are foods you shop for regularly.

The pantry also includes on-the-go foods that are a part of our mobile culture. Having healthy versions of snacks helps maintain a healthy lifestyle! This type of pre-planning can ward off unwanted food temptations, because when we're hungry, we eat what's handy. Make sure that what you have handy is also healthy. Remember, we are what we eat!

PANTRY ORGANIZATION

Having an organized pantry is a great habit to cultivate—order sets the mind at ease and allows you to be in control of your food choices. With a well-planned pantry, your kitchen will function more effectively, so let's talk about pantry organization. The keys to a well-planned pantry are accessibility and visibility, meaning knowing what you have on hand and being able to retrieve the items you want quickly. The time invested in organizing your pantry will be returned many times over as you enjoy healthy eating.

Easy steps for organizing your pantry:

1. Declutter
    - Empty pantry items out onto a counter or surface.
    - Check the expiration dates.
    - Sort and categorize the rest by food type.
    - Inventory what you have and decide what to keep.
    - Toss out undesirable and expired food items.

1a. Debug (a.k.a. pantry pest management)
    - Most dried food products are susceptible to insect infestation (especially flour, baking mixes, packaged foods, crackers, spices and powdered milk)
    - **Beware** of dry goods in plastic or paper bags! These are particularly susceptible.

    Suggested storage options:
    - Store in glass: use mason jars or re-use glass containers
    - Store flour, grains, nuts and seeds in the refrigerator for short-term storage
    - Store flour, grains, nuts and seeds in the freezer for long-term storage

2. Create your pantry item list. Use the list to identify, restock, "and "add new pantry items.

3. Select a storage arrangement that suits your lifestyle, such as:
    a. Pantry items just placed together, period.
    b. Pantry items placed together and organized by:
        - Categories: spices, baking goods, grains, etc.
        - Areas: items grouped in the following way:
            - ***Morning/breakfast area:*** Cereals, oats, protein bars, etc.
            - ***Dinner area:*** Couscous, quinoa, dry beans, etc.
            - ***Children's area*** (i.e., reachable by children):
                - Healthy snacks
                - Nut butters (almond, cashew, sunflower seed, etc.)
                - Popcorn
                - Sunflower seed

    If space is limited, use the minimalist approach: spare and streamline

PANTRY ITEMS FOR RECIPES

BAKING GOODS
Arrowroot flour
Baking powder (aluminum free)
Baking soda
Buckwheat flour
Cornmeal, organic
Coconut sugar
Maple Syrup
Raw Agave Nectar
Spelt flour

CONDIMENTS
BBQ Sauce
Celtic Sea Salt
Mustard, Coarse Grain

CAN/JAR/ PAKAGED FOODS
Artichokes (marinated)
Beans/Legumes (or fresh)
Chickpea pasta
Coconut Milk
Molasses
Relish (sweet)
Soba Noodles, buckwheat
Tahini Paste
Tomatoes (whole, diced, paste)
Vinegar (apple cider, balsamic)

GRAINS
Einkorn (wheatberries)
Oats, Old Fashion rolled
Quinoa (white, red)
Wild Rice

NUTS & SEEDS
Almonds
Cashews
Walnuts
Chia seeds
Flax seeds
Mustard seeds (yellow)
Pumpkin seeds (pepita)
Sesame Seeds (black, tan)
Sunflower seeds

OIL
Coconut oil (unrefined)
Flaxseed oil (no heat)
Olive oil (extra virgin)
Walnut oil

MISCELLANOUS
Cacao Powder
Dried fruit/flowers (apricots, cranberries,
dates, raisins) hibiscus petals
Garlic
Kalamata Olives (also in jars)
Nutritional Yeast
Pure Vanilla Extract

HERBS & SPICES
See Herbs and Spices, page 41

REFRIGERATOR: COLD STORAGE

A clean, fresh refrigerator is a supportive resource to help you meet healthy lifestyle goals, including: quicker meal preparation, less spoilage, less wasted food, improved health and whatever else you deem to be important to you and your family.

A refrigerator is a cold storage pantry and much more. Properly storing food in the refrigerator and freezer is often minimized and overlooked, yet it is a significant part of an orderly kitchen and your new healthy eating lifestyle. While nonperishable packaged foods will stay fresh for a month or more in a regular pantry, refrigerated foods—especially plant foods—have a much shorter shelf life. Knowing which foods should be refrigerated can save you money, prevent food spoilage and possible food poisoning.

FOODS BEST REFRIGERATED	FOODS BEST NOT REFRIGERATED
Apples	Bananas
Citrus fruits (lemons, limes)	Garlic, onion
Condiments once opened	Olive Oil
Leafy greens (lettuce, spinach)	Potatoes
Nuts and seeds	Stone fruit (peaches, plums)
Plant/nut milk	Tomatoes
Produce (celery, carrots, cabbage, beets)	Whole winter squash (acorn, butternut, etc.)

To receive maximum return on your food investments, these practices can make a difference:

- Wipe out the refrigerator before shopping (weekly or biweekly).
- Toss away or compost any expired/perished foods.
- Get produce home in a timely matter.
- Do not leave perishable foods in hot car or in a sunny spot.
- Separate special item- like lettuce and leafy greens are best washed just before preparing.

- Most fresh produce should be eaten within 3-5 days, but when stored properly, it can last longer.
- Rotate produce: use produce that has already been in the refrigerator first, then use newly purchased produce.

Keeping produce chilled slows down its metabolic activity. Vegetables and fruits that need to be refrigerated are best stored at refrigerator temperatures of 30° to 50°F (-1° to 4°C). Also, limiting exposure to oxygen reduces tissue breakdown, or oxidation. This is often accomplished by storing produce in airtight containers. Airtight containers also protect fruits and vegetables from excess moisture. Since most fruits and vegetables are 70% to 95% water, excess moisture will cause them to become wilted and limp. Excess moisture also causes mold growth and rot.

Moisture in lettuce and leafy greens should be removed by gently placing the leaves on a towel and patting them dry or using a salad spinner. We want to work with salad greens that are dry. This helps the dressing cling to the leaves, especially if you're using a delicate green like lettuce. With a sturdier green like kale, swiss chard, or arugula, we still want to start with bone-dry greens to reduce the risk of having a soggy salad. Store unused dry leaves in a plastic bag to be used within a couple days. When placing vegetables or fruit in a plastic bag, gently squeeze out all the air before closing the bag. You can also vacuum-seal the bag by closing it and leaving a small space into which you insert a straw. Use the straw to suck out all the air, then quickly remove the straw and close the bag. Store ripening fruit at room temperature. This allows the fruit to breathe. To hasten the ripening process of any fruit, store it in a paper bag at room temperature.

ETHYLENE IN FRUITS AND VEGETABLES

Ethylene is a gas released by some fruits and vegetables that cause produce to ripen faster. Some fruits and vegetables are more sensitive to ethylene than others. Correct storage of fruits and vegetables can reduce food waste. Below are ethylene sensitive and ethylene producers:

Ethylene Sensitive fruits and vegetables:
Apples · Asparagus · Avocados · Bananas · Broccoli · Cantaloupe · Collard Greens Cucumber · Eggplant · Grapes · Honeydew · Kiwi · Lemons · Lettuce · Limes · Mangoes Onions · Peaches · Pears · Peppers · Squash · Sweet Potatoes · Watermelon

Ethylene Producers:
Apples · Avocados · Bananas · Cantaloupe · Kiwi · Peaches· Pears · Peppers · Tomatoes

Do not store fruits and vegetables that produce ethylene with those that are sensitive to ethylene. For example, do not store bananas and apples next to each other. This applies to produce that is refrigerated and not refrigerated.

Note: The above sections written by Beverly Flemings and have been medically reviewed by Registered Dietitian Nutritionist, Erin Beattie. www.Thriving-Health.com.

REFRIGERATOR ORGANIZATION

A fresh refrigerator is an amazingly culinary resource! Set up your refrigerator and maintain your cold storage pantry with whatever system you choose. There is a growing variety of organizing systems (products) of every size and shape to help you access and maintain your refrigerated items! Most of the products are wonderful and handy. Then again, you may already have products in your home that will assist you. The organizing process begins with you and your goals. Organizing products alone will not organize you—they are only an accessory or tool to help you maintain order.

Here's how to bring order to the refrigerator:

- Empty items onto a counter or surface.
- Check labels for expiration dates and examine perishables for freshness.
- Toss out expired items and old food.
- Sort and categorize foods by their type.

- Clear, clean, and wipe the refrigerator out.
    - Do a quarterly refrigerator clean of the inside and outside
- Store plant foods properly to maintain freshness.
    - **Note:** Most greens are best washed right before use!
    - Keep nuts, seeds, grains, and flour in the crisper or freezer.

In order to facilitate your cold pantry storage even more, let's talk about the different temperature zones inside of an average refrigerator.

REFRIGERATOR TEMPERATURE ZONES

Modern refrigerators have different temperature zones. These different zones allow food to be properly stored so that it doesn't spoil. When food is properly chilled, growth of bacteria and other microbes is prohibited. The refrigerator keeps perishable items fresh for a short time, while the freezer is for long-term food storage.

When refrigerating food, it helps to understand what a "short" period of time is. Since produce usually doesn't come with an expiration date. It is important to have a rotation system in place for fresh produce. "Rotating" means remembering when you put a particular piece of produce in the refrigerator and rotating it to the front when you buy another of that same produce. For example, prepare the fresh collards you purchased last Saturday before preparing the collards you purchased today. You might want to post a whiteboard on the side of the refrigerator to track this information. Make it as easy on your brain as possible!

Placing foods in the appropriate temperate zones is how foods in cold storage are maintained.

Let's look at the temperature zones of an average refrigerator:

- The warmest area of the refrigerator are shelves built into the doors. Great to store condiments.
- The most consistent temperature is on the top shelf.

- The middle shelf where the eye goes first is ideal for leftovers and foods you want to see.
- The coldest temperature is the bottom shelf, making it great for eggs and meat.
- The crisper has high humidity and is ideal for leafy greens and other produce.
- **Note:** Raw nuts, whole grains, seeds, and flours can also be kept in the refrigerator or freezer to greatly extend their life.

Properly storing and consuming fresh food is a great benefit of natural eating.

QUICK TIPS FOR ORGANIZING YOUR REFRIGERATOR

- Store like items together. (storing all condiments together; beverages together, etc.)
- Organize refrigerator contents to clearly view what's inside when you first open it.
- Avoid overloading the refrigerator—the cold air needs room to circulate.
- Pre-prep food when time is an issue and keep it refrigerated until needed.
- Store new duplicate products directly behind already-open products.
- Keep the refrigerator fresh with an opened box of Arm & Hammer baking soda. This will last for 3 months.

THE FREEZER AND FROZEN FOODS

Below are tips to save you money and food waste. Label frozen foods with the date and description of the food.

- Keep a running food inventory, updating food as it's added and removed.
    - Consider an erasable marker and whiteboard/clipboard attached close to the refrigerator.
- Defrost regularly, i.e., when ¼" of ice appears.
- When filling freezer bags with soups, sauces, and other foods that can be stored as a flat single layer, squeeze out the excess air and then freeze flat. This will enable you to stack flat-frozen foods on top of each other to maximize your freezer space.
- Store like foods together (veggies together; soups and stews together, etc.)
- Use freezer containers and baskets to help organize your frozen goods.

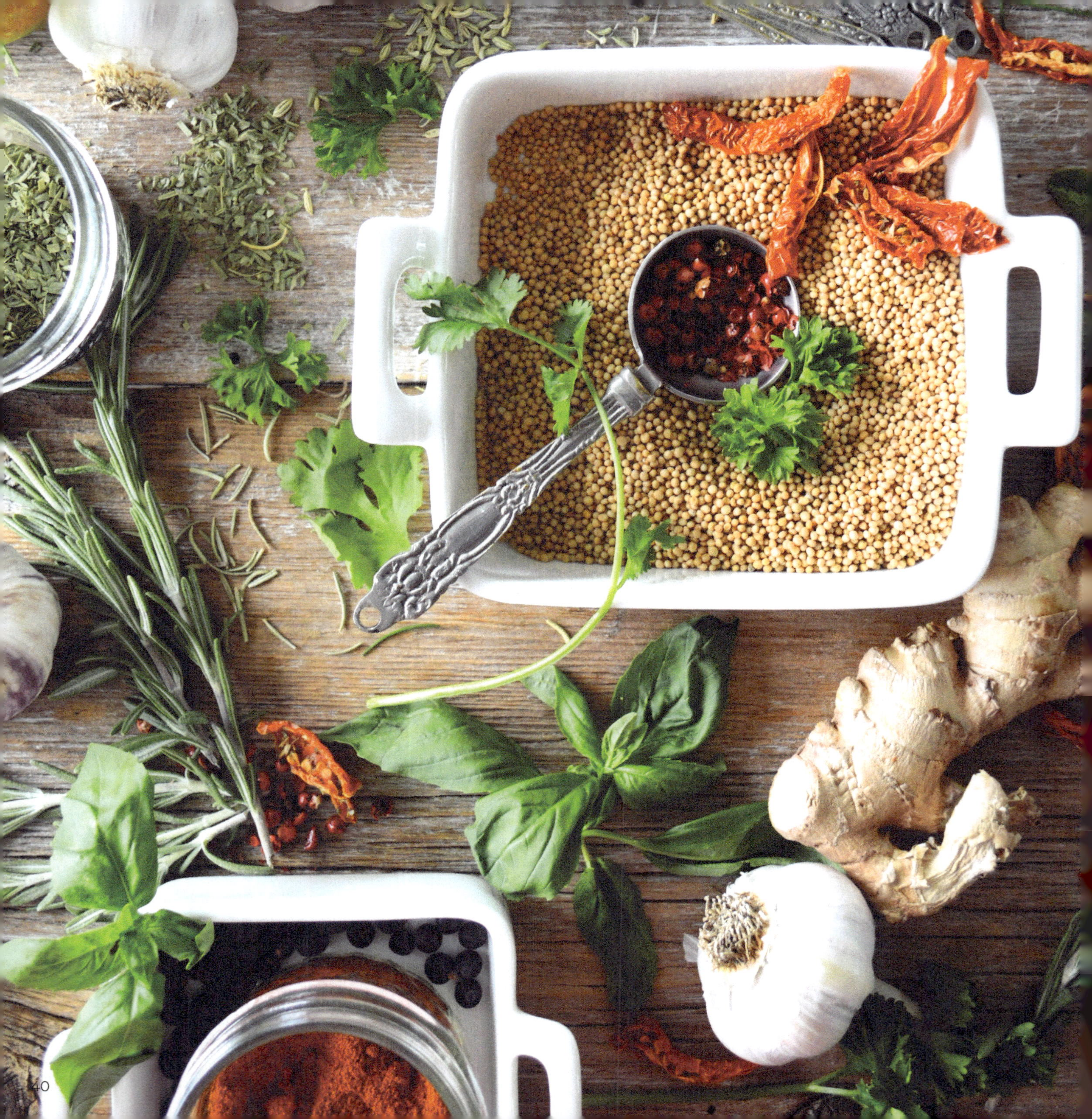

HERBS AND SPICES

An element of the lifestyle change is recognizing that plant-based eating, is eating from the earth – for real. Leaving the world of process foods and entering nature's domain will open you to a more advance world of food options and health options.
By using herbs, spices, and other seasonings your food is dramatically transformed and thus, your palate. Herbs and spices boost the flavor of home cooked food and can heighten the nutritional profile of dishes. Adding fresh herbs, dried herbs and ground spices, gives food a greater depth of flavor and texture. It also reduces the urge to overcompensate with salt.

Since dried herbs supply more concentrated flavor than fresh herbs. When substituting fresh herbs for dried herbs in a recipe, the rule of thumb is to use 3 times as much of the fresh as their dried counterpart. Herbs come from the leaves, seeds, and flowers of plants, and are available fresh and dried. Spices come from the bark, buds, fruit, root, or stems of various trees and plants, and are available whole (to grind) or ground in powdered form.

Historically, herbs were introduced as medicine; before they were used in cooking. The medicinal properties of many herbs contribute to their presence (or carryover) in our kitchen today. As people trusted to believe that a particular herb was helpful to their health need, they begin to infuse herbs into their food. and into their body

Working with herbs and spices is learning flavors and tastes, most of all learning about your preferences and enjoying the process that leads to Good eats!

Allspice – also known as Jamaica Pepper, is native to the West Indies and Central America. Has a mixture of Cinnamon, Nutmeg and Cloves in taste.

Basil – a sweet, flavorful, leafy green herb. Delicate and delicious to eat fresh; when cut lasts 3-5 days.

Bay Leaves – the dried whole leaves are added to slow-cooking recipes (soups, sauces, stews) and must be removed before serving the dish.

Black Pepper – a spice made by grinding dry Peppercorns. Has a sharp, mildly spicy flavor that goes well with many dishes. Known as the "king of spices" it has been used for thousands of years.

Cardamom – a herb with a very strong, sweet pungent flavor and aroma. Whole pods, easily crushed, are used in Lentil recipes; is an essential ingredient in Indian, Middle Eastern and Nordic cuisine.

Cayenne Pepper – is available in dry pods or powder form. The active ingredient, capsaicin, is "moderately hot" in this chili pepper. Has an impressive nutritional profile including antioxidants.

Chicory Root – in its dry/ground form contains inulin which accounts for its bitter taste.

Chili Powder – a red-colored blend of powdered spices. Usually contains Cayenne Pepper for heat, but also Cumin, Garlic Powder, Oregano and Paprika, depending on the blend.

Cinnamon (ground & stick) – a spice from the bark of Cinnamon trees. The sweet, warming aroma and flavor derive from its oil. Used in history dating back to Ancient Egypt.

Cloves – a pungent spice used in savory dishes, desserts and drinks. Mainly used in Asian, African, Mediterranean and Middle East countries in curries, marinades, and more.

Coriander – referred to as both an herb and a spice. Fresh coriander is called by its Mexican name cilantro. Dried seed is the coriander seed. Used to flavor Mediterranean and Middle East recipes.

Crushed Red Pepper or Red Pepper Flakes - a spice consisting of dried and crushed Red Chili Peppers; adds fiery fresh heat and a zesty flavor boost to any recipe.

Cumin – a earthy, warm spice used in Latin American, North African, Middle Eastern and Indian cuisines. Available both as whole seeds and in ground form.

Curry Powder – a mixture of dried, ground spices of a yellow or orange hue; sweet pungency. Usually contains Turmeric, Cumin, Ginger, Black Pepper, may also contain Garlic and Cinnamon.

Dandelion Root – a herb; when roasted, is a popular coffee alternative which doesn't contain caffeine; can be made into teas, etc. Has an impressive list of health benefits.

Garam Masala – a blend of ground spices: Cumin, Coriander, Cardamom, Black Pepper, Cinnamon, Cloves, Nutmeg. Is traditionally used throughout India

---

Ginger – has been an important spice for more than 3,000 years. It has a tangy flavor with a bite. Ginger and Garlic are natural flavor partners. Ground or fresh, only a little is needed to flavor a recipe.

Ground Chili – a ground powder made of Chili Peppers; used by spice lovers all over the world it gives an intense kick to recipes. Comes in a variety of "hot" levels from mild to super-fiery.

Mustard Seeds – a spice, tiny yellow, brown or black; have a faint spicy smell. Used for pickling, making mustard, other condiments, also in curries, sauces to give a pungent, slightly spicy flavor.

Nutmeg – a spice from fragrant evergreen tree where two spices, mace and nutmeg, grow together in the same fruit. Nutmeg has a pungent fragrance and deep woody taste. A little goes a long way.

Onion Powder – is dehydrated, ground Onion; is found in spice mixes. Being more commonly used now.

Oregano – a herb; strong aroma and slightly bitter, earthy flavor. Commonly used in Italian dishes.

Rosemary – a herb; the leaves are fragrant, woody, aromatic, with a slightly bitter taste; used dried or fresh in recipes.

Smoked Paprika – is considered a "gourmet" spice; has a smoky, woodsy, spicy flavor. Made by slowly smoking Paprika Peppers over oak wood.

Thyme – a herb; used to season all kinds of dishes; a pleasant, pungent, clover flavor; can be consumed fresh or dried. Adds a savory note to soups, veggie burgers and vegetables.

Turmeric – a spice; has a warm, woodsy taste, floral, citrus and a slightly bitter taste; commonly used to flavor or color curry powders, mustards, and in rich stew sauces.

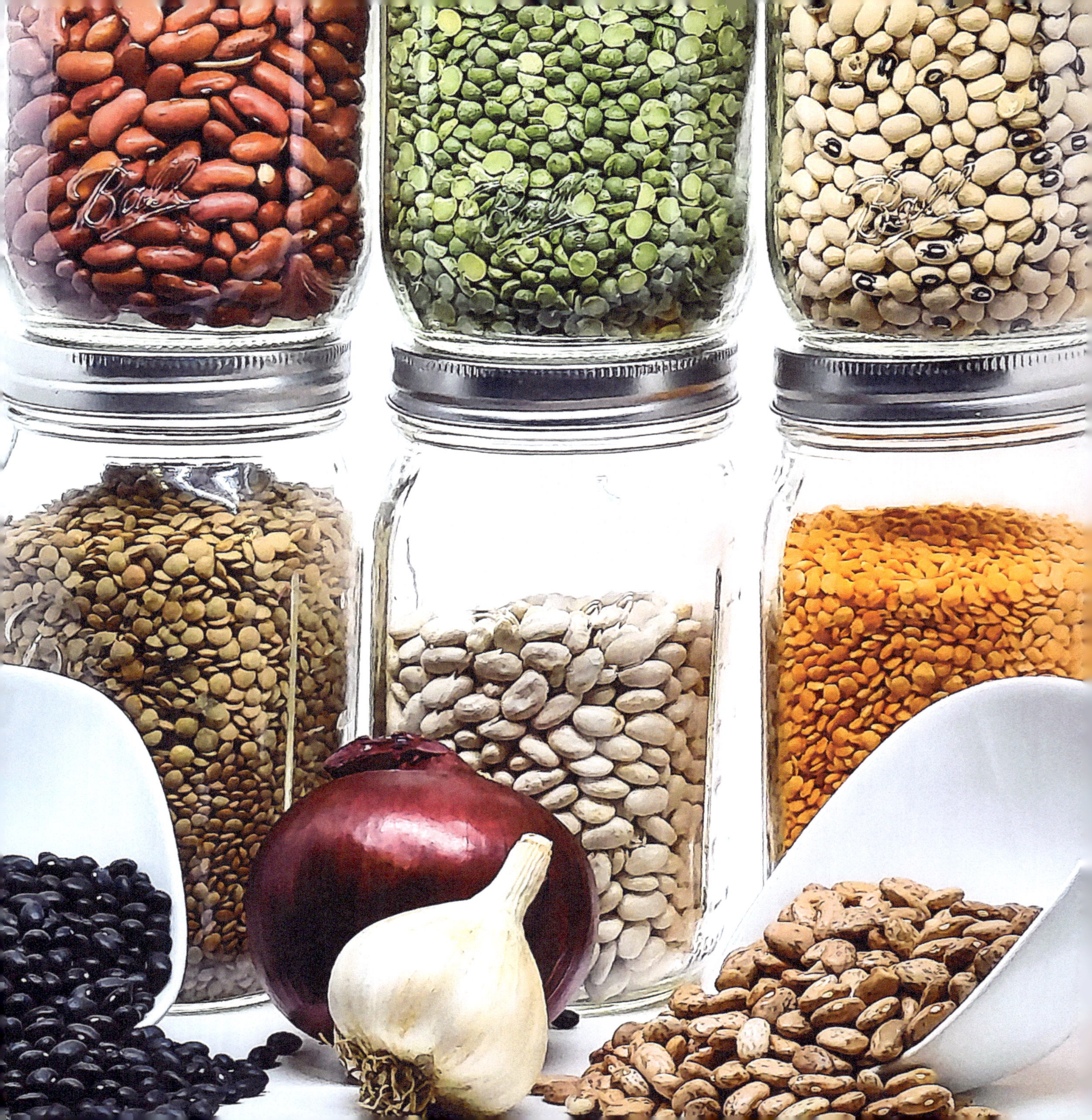

LEGUMES

Legumes are the foundation of cuisine the world over and include beans, peas, and lentils. They are low glycemic foods very rich in minerals, vitamins and full of fiber. Beans are among the highest protein content of all plant foods. Beans contain antioxidants, vitamins and minerals, such as iron, magnesium, phosphorous, potassium and zinc. Beans and lentils from an organic farmer can give you a whole new bean experience.

The variety of beans and legumes is vast enough to satisfy any palate. The more popular varieties: red beans, navy beans, black beans, azuki beans, lima beans, fava beans, pinto beans, black eyed peas, and chickpeas. Red lentils, green and brown lentils, French Lentils, and Black Beluga lentils. If your intake of nutrients fall short of the daily dietary allowance, beans and legumes could be/ can be a great source to refuel your body.

Canned beans are convenient and great to keep on hand, but dried beans are more nutritious and lower in sodium. One pound of dried beans (2 cups) will make 5 - 6 cups of cooked beans.

How To Cook Dried Beans –

Select the freshest product possible. Sort and remove any debris before rinsing. I suggest soaking dried beans, except black-eyed peas, overnight. Discard soaking water before cooking.

Soak beans before cooking to: a) reduce the cooking time. b) release the bean starch c) lessen the gas releasing properties d) decrease phytic acid.

1. Sauté aromatics (onions, garlic, celery, carrots) in a little oil to add flavor and aroma.
2. Add fresh water, beans and bay leaves to a medium pot and bring to a boil, reduce heat to simmer.
3. Stir every 30 minutes to ensure there is no sticking and enough water is available.

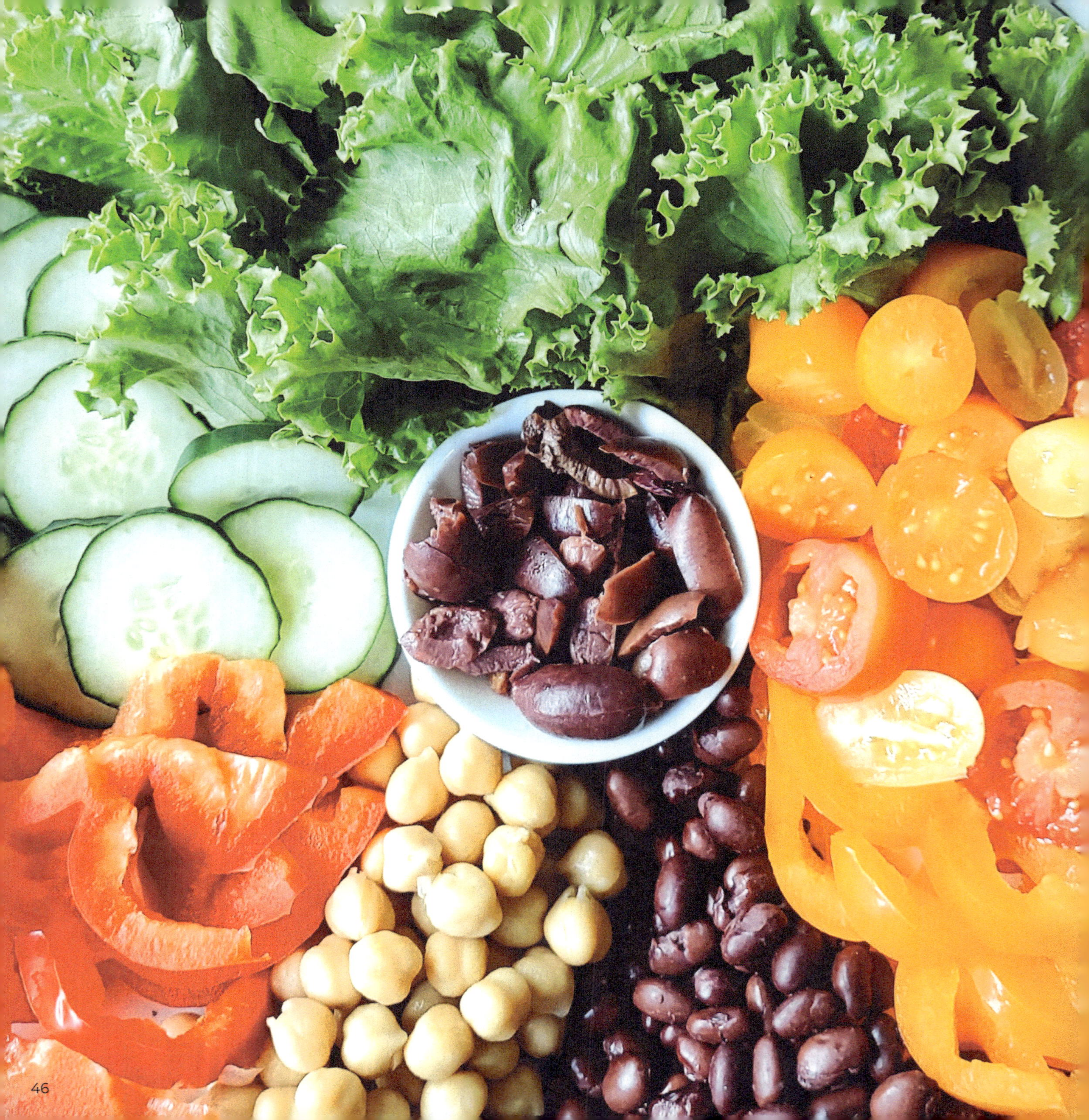

Recipes

Part Two

Spring Vegetables and Fruits

(partial listing)

Arugula

Asparagus

Bok Choy

Carrots

Dandelion Greens

Fennel

Green Garlic

Leeks

Mustard Greens

Nettle

Radishes

Rhubarb

Spinach

Spring Mix

Spring Onions

Swiss Chard

Turnip Greens

Avocado

Kiwi

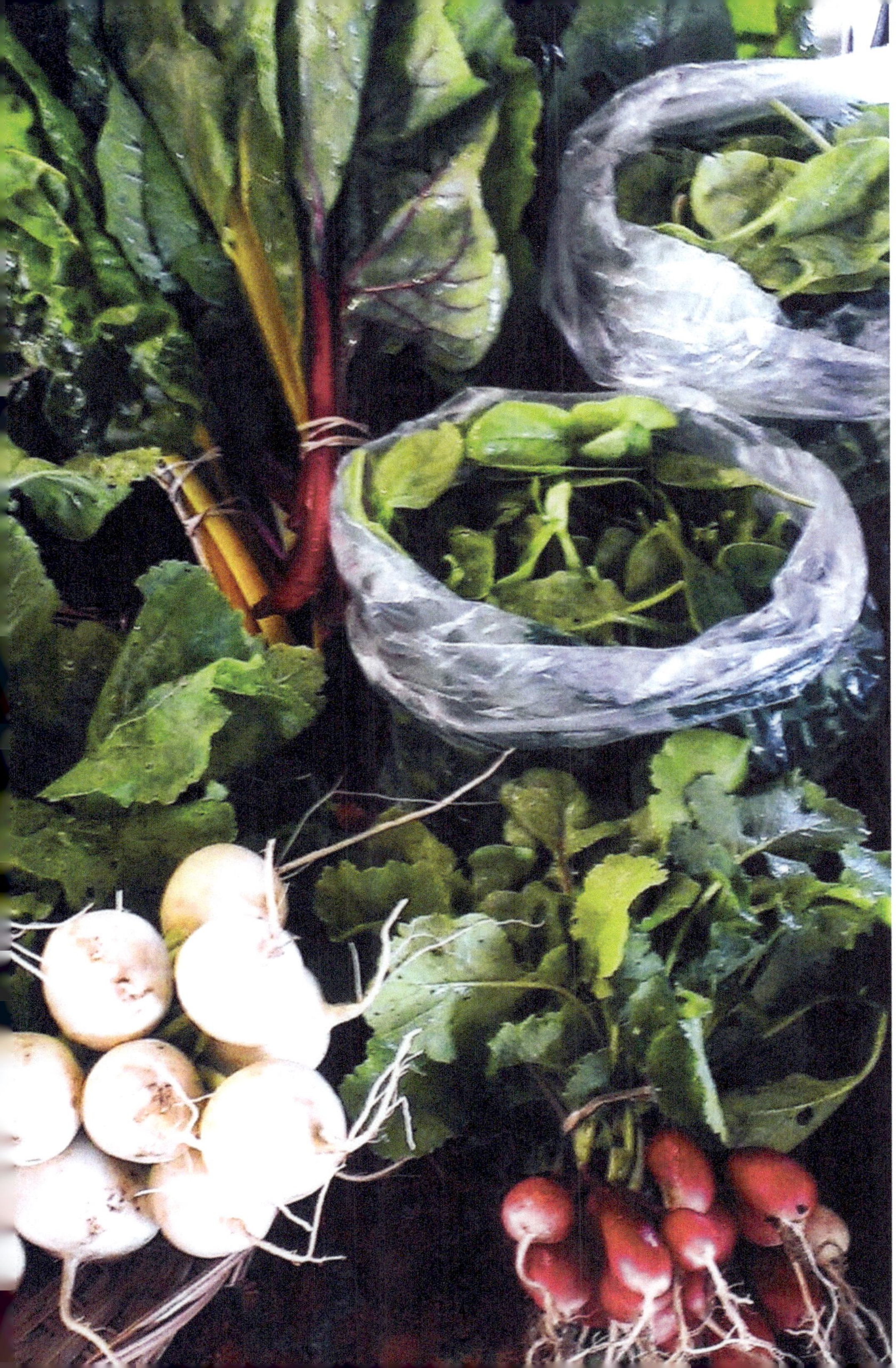

SPRING

MARCH, APRIL + MAY

SPRING RECIPES

Spring's arrival brings renewal, rebirth, and new beginnings. It's time for spring cleaning and for opening windows to bring fresh air into our homes. Just as our home needs a spring cleaning, so does our body. Decluttering begins the process to reclaim space and create clarity.

A spring detox can regenerate the body's systems, help clear out toxins that accumulate over the winter months, and rid the body of a lethargic feeling. Spring detoxification can play a vital role in overall health maintenance. It is important to consciously support our detoxifying, i.e., the liver and kidneys. Detoxification can be a natural process as early spring plants like those in the salads that follow are consumed. Fresh herbs, wild greens, and bitter greens grow naturally at this time of the year. These plants are a vital part of the seasonal landscape and are nature's pharmacy.

Spring is the time to indulge in delicate first of the season produce, so this section largely features seasonal greens. For me, the highlight of the spring season is returning to the farmers' markets, welcoming the farmers back, and purchasing their fresh, seasonal foods. Early spring offerings also include a variety of tender baby lettuces and hearty greens like baby arugula, baby mustard greens, baby spinach, baby kale and chard. It's highly likely that you will also find bitter greens like dandelion and possibly nettle. Bitter greens are essentially absent from the modern American diet, but are important for healthy digestion, for absorbing certain vitamins, and for strengthening tissues.

The early spring season also produces an array of crisp, nutritious Asian greens like tatsoi, mizuna komatsuna, and bok choy. As we move into late spring, tender green garlic will be on the scene, along with nutrient-rich sunflower shoots, sweet pea shoots, and microgreens. Microgreens are not to be confused with bean sprouts—they are not the same. Microgreens are a powerhouse of nutrition and flavor and can be consumed raw in a salad, lightly sautéed, or used in smoothies.

Let's welcome spring!

FRESH SPRING PEA SOUP

It's spring and sweet peas are in season— what a great time to flow with the season! A pot of fresh sweet pea soup is filling, delicious, and super quick to prepare. Sweet peas are a rich source of minerals and vitamin B. Smaller peas tend to be sweeter.

INGREDIENTS:

1 ½ cups vegetable broth
1 small onion, chopped
2 cloves garlic, minced
2 cups sweet peas, or one 12-ounce bag frozen sweet peas
Leaves from 10 mint sprigs (a sprig is 3 or more leaves on a stem)
One 15-ounce can of light coconut milk
1 ½ teaspoons fresh lemon juice
1/2 teaspoon Celtic sea salt

PREPARATION:

1. In a large soup pot over medium heat, warm vegetable broth. Add onions and garlic and cook for 5 minutes.

2. Stir in peas, mint leaves, and coconut milk. Reduce heat to low and simmer for 5 minutes. Turn the heat off and allow to cool.

3. Once cool, place ingredients in a blender. Add lemon juice and salt (omit salt for low-salt diets) and blend until smooth. Taste and add extra water as desired.

Makes 32 ounces

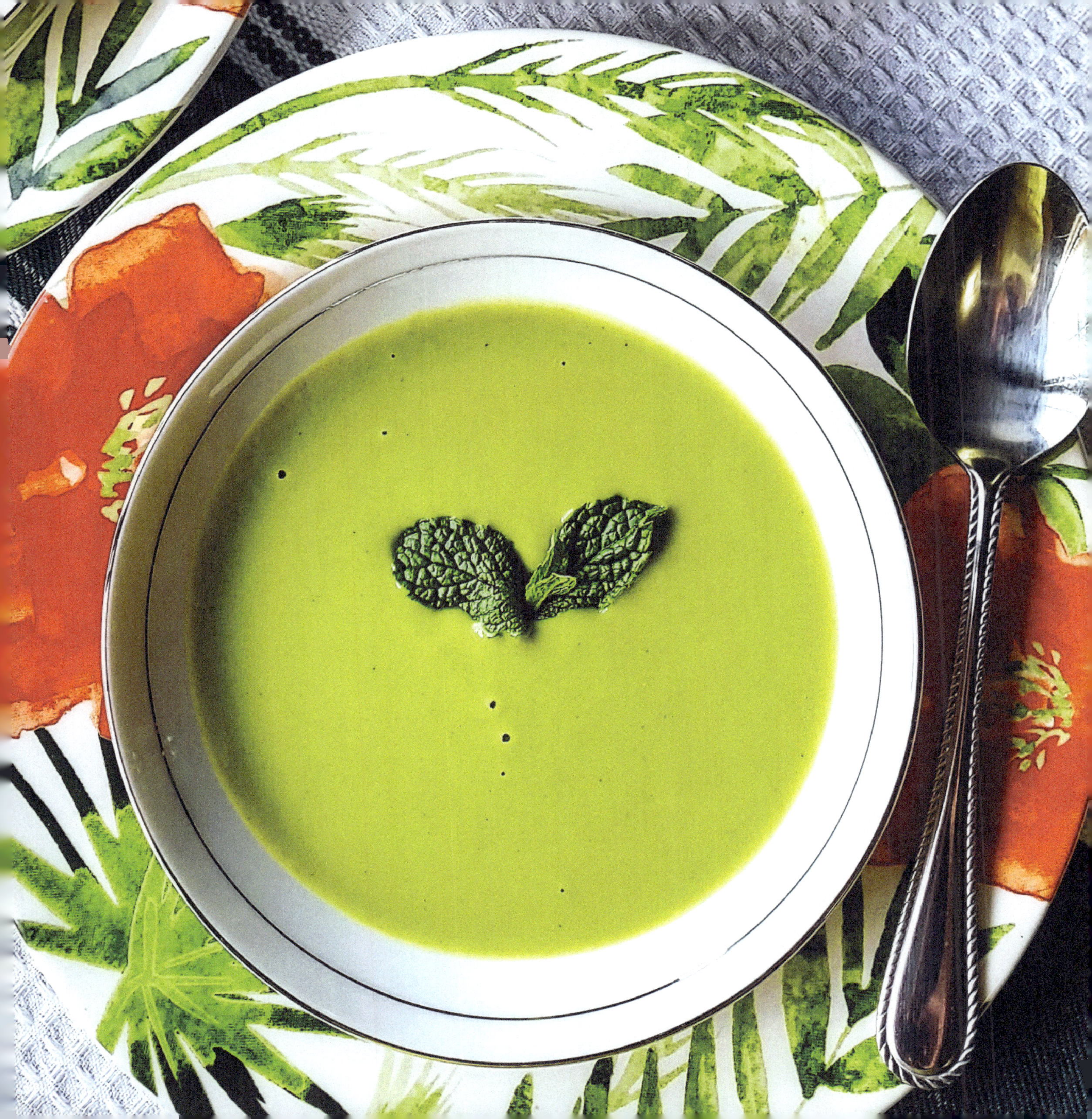

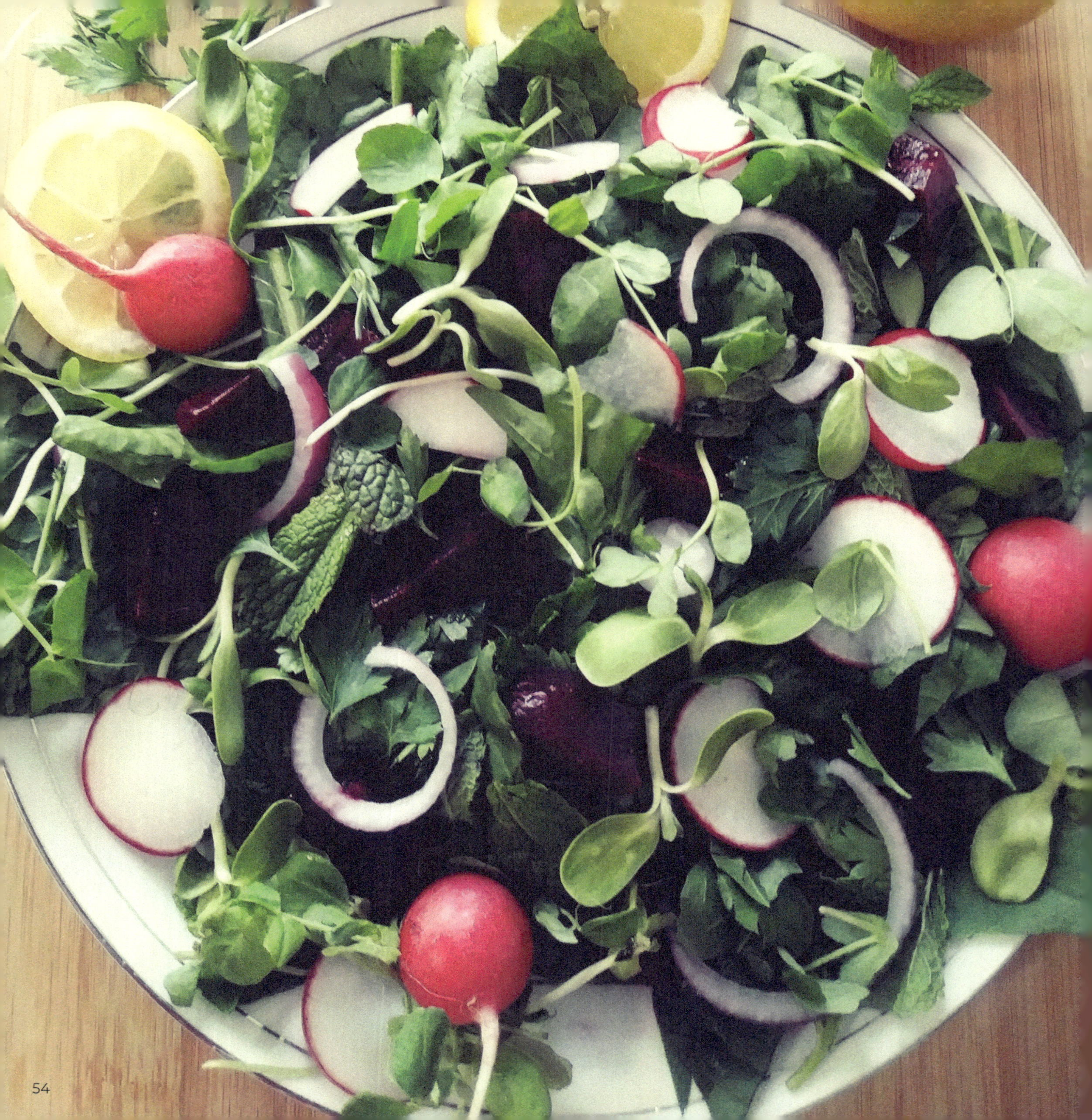

SPRING SALAD WITH FRESH HERBS

Throughout the spring season, we're seeing green again and again. This salad with fresh herbs is spring in a bowl — I've mixed together spring greens, some fresh herbs, and radishes. Radishes add crispiness, spice, and crunch, plus they are a great source of antioxidants. Allow this recipe to be a template for more salads!

INGREDIENTS:
2 cups spring mix
1 ½ cups dandelion leaves, chopped (young leaves, preferably)
1 medium purple beet
2 cups fresh herb leaves (basil, mint, or herbs of your choice)
4 radishes, trimmed and sliced
1 cup of sunflower shoots
Tahini-Lime Dressing

Tahini-Lime Dressing - Makes ½ cup
4 tablespoons tahini paste
4 tablespoons water
4 tablespoons fresh lime juice
1 teaspoon ground ginger
2 teaspoon whole grain mustard *(see recipe page. 196)*
1 tablespoon honey

PREPARATION: For all greens: wash and spin dry.

1. Prepare beet: Remove beet greens (trim away ½" of the beet stem, retain the tail). Place beet in medium-size saucepan, cover with water, and bring to a boil. Reduce heat and simmer until beet is tender to the touch of a fork (approximately 35 minutes). Drain and cool.

2. While the beets are cooking:
   Make the Tahini -Lime Dressing - place all ingredients in a blender and blend until smooth. To thin the consistency, add small amounts of water, until you reach desired taste. Leftover dressing will last 5 days in refrigerator.

3. The beet skin will slip off easily when cool. Cut beet in half, into quarters, then into wedges.

4. Place spring mix, dandelions, and herbs in large salad bowl and toss to blend. Portion the greens into 4 salad bowls.

5. Add beets and radishes to each bowl and top with sunflower sprouts.

6. Serve with Tahini-Lime Dressing.

Makes 4 servings

SPRING DANDELION - CITRUS SALAD

Dandelion leaves are among the first greens of the season. Spring dandelion leaves are full of the essential minerals potassium, calcium, and magnesium. They are less bitter than their autumn counterparts and are also a great source of protein, fiber, and antioxidants. When I saw a ripe pineapple, my mind clicked and voilà! This recipe was the result: a gentle spring detox.

INGREDIENTS:

3 cups Swiss chard leaves (4 small or 2 large leaves), stems removed
½ bunch organic dandelion leaves (approximately 14 leaves), trimmed
1 ½ cups fresh pineapple, cut into chunks
2 oranges
1 medium avocado, cubed
Juice of ½ lemon
Handful of pepita (pumpkin) seeds
Optional: Sesame seeds (1 tablespoon)

PREPARATION:

1. Wash, spin, and then dry the Swiss chard leaves. Roll them into tight cylinders. Cut into ribbons and then cut diagonally.
2. Chop the dandelion leaves. Squeeze the juice from 1 orange and set aside. Peel the other orange and segment it, then coarsely chop the segments.
3. In a large salad bowl, place the greens, pineapple chunks, orange segments, and avocado cubes.
4. Combine the orange juice and lemon juice. Pour the juice over the salad and toss to coat the wilted greens. Sprinkle pepita seeds on top. Sesame seeds are also an option.

Makes 4 servings

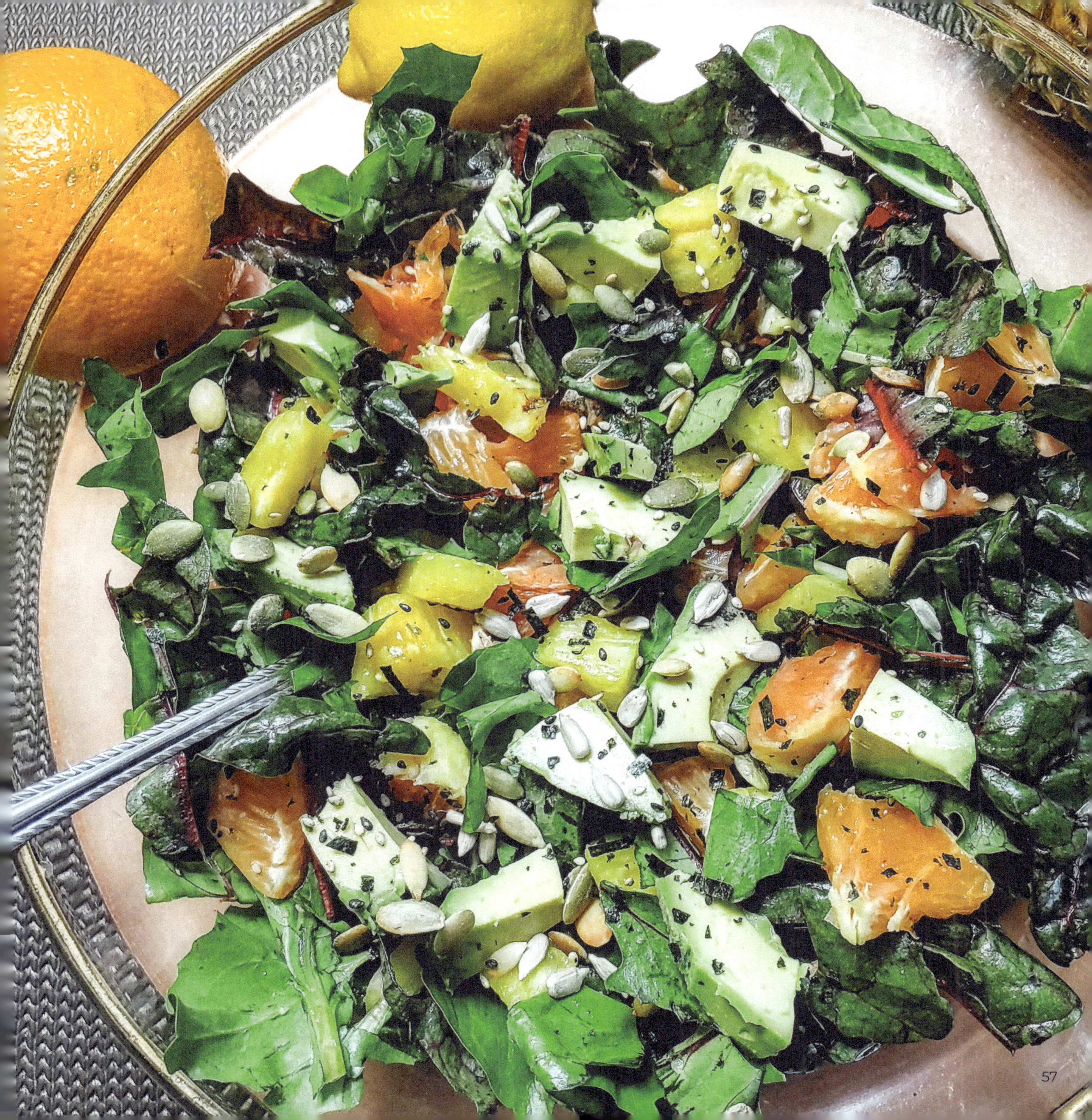

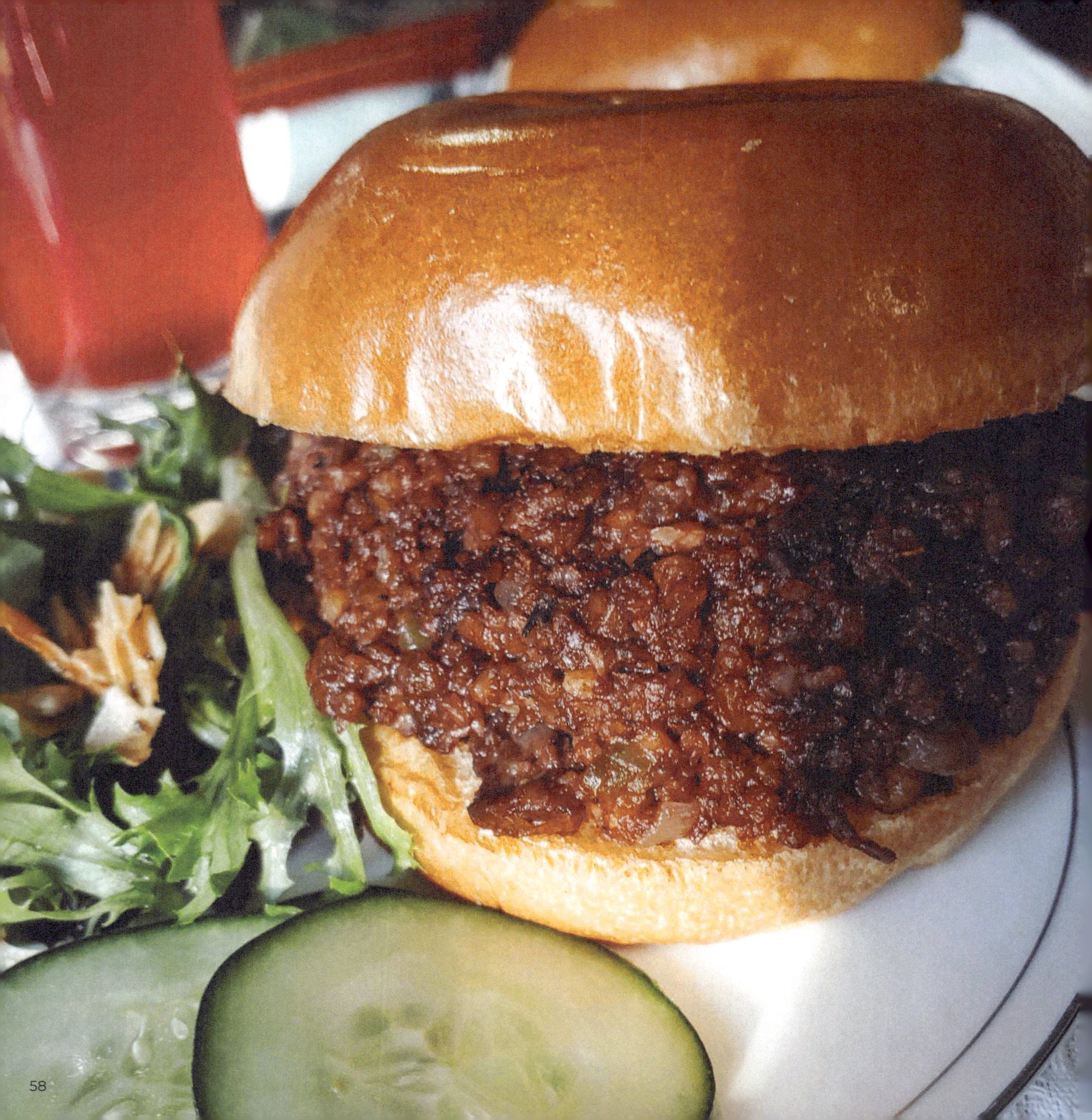

SLOPPY JOE "NUT" BURGERS

This recipe is my favorite rendition of the classic Sloppy Joe burger. I originally created it in the 1970s so my children would not feel left out when their friends were eating their traditional Sloppy Joe burgers. It has stood the test of time.

INGREDIENTS:

1 cup (½ pound) raw cashews, soaked for 6 hours and then drained (reserve the soaking liquid)
2 tablespoons olive oil
1 small onion, chopped
3 cloves garlic, minced
1 green bell pepper, diced
½ teaspoon dried oregano
½ teaspoon dried thyme
½ teaspoon ground sage
½ teaspoon smoked paprika
1 teaspoon ground cumin
1 teaspoon Celtic sea salt
Dash of cayenne pepper
2 ½ tablespoons BBQ sauce (see page 200)
4 buns

PREPARATION:

Note: The cashews must be dry! If they are too wet, they will not grind properly.

1. Wrap the soaked cashews in a kitchen towel to absorb any water, then spread the cashews out to dry thoroughly. Grind the dried cashews in a food processor until they become a coarse meal. Set aside.

2. Warm the olive oil in a large skillet over medium-low heat. Add onion and garlic and sauté for 2 minutes. Stir in the green pepper and the cashew mixture. If the mixture is to dry to stir, pour in some of the reserved soaking liquid from the cashews.

3. Remove from heat and stir in the herbs, spices, salt and pepper. Return the skillet to low heat and add the barbecue sauce. If the mixture still needs to be "sloppier," add more of the reserved soaking liquid. Serve on buns.

Makes 4 servings

QUINOA GREEN DINNER SALAD

This quinoa green salad offers one of the best combination within the food kingdom. Its foundation is quinoa, which contains all nine essential amino acids, making quinoa a complete plant protein.

Swiss chard greens provide a superb source of potassium, magnesium, and protein. The citrus dressing lifts all of the flavors in this salad. I trust you will enjoy this salad as much as I do!

Note: The salad is best when the quinoa is prepared a day prior.

SALAD INGREDIENTS:

3 cups red Swiss chard (organic when possible), washed and stems removed
1 cup cooked quinoa, prepared a day prior*
½ red bell pepper, finely diced
2 green onions, sliced thin
1 rib celery, finely diced
2 carrots, finely diced
1 cup dried unsweetened cranberries
¼ cup walnuts, chopped

DRESSING INGREDIENTS:

1 teaspoon ground ginger
Juice of 1 orange
½ teaspoon fresh lime juice
1 tablespoon flaxseed oil
1 tablespoon walnut oil or olive oil
Celtic sea salt and pepper to taste

PREPARATION:

The dressing: Whisk together the ingredients.

The salad:

1. Stack the Swiss chard leaves, roll lengthwise into tight cylinders or tubes. Slice across the tubes, producing ribbons and then cut the ribbons diagonally.

2. Place cooked quinoa in a large bowl and fluff with a fork. Add the red pepper, green onions, celery and carrots. Drizzle the dressing over the quinoa, small amounts at a time so not to saturate and toss to mix.

3. Add the chopped Swiss chard. Toss well to combine all ingredients, then add the cranberries and walnuts. Store any leftover dressing in airtight container in the refrigerator.

Makes 4 to 6 servings

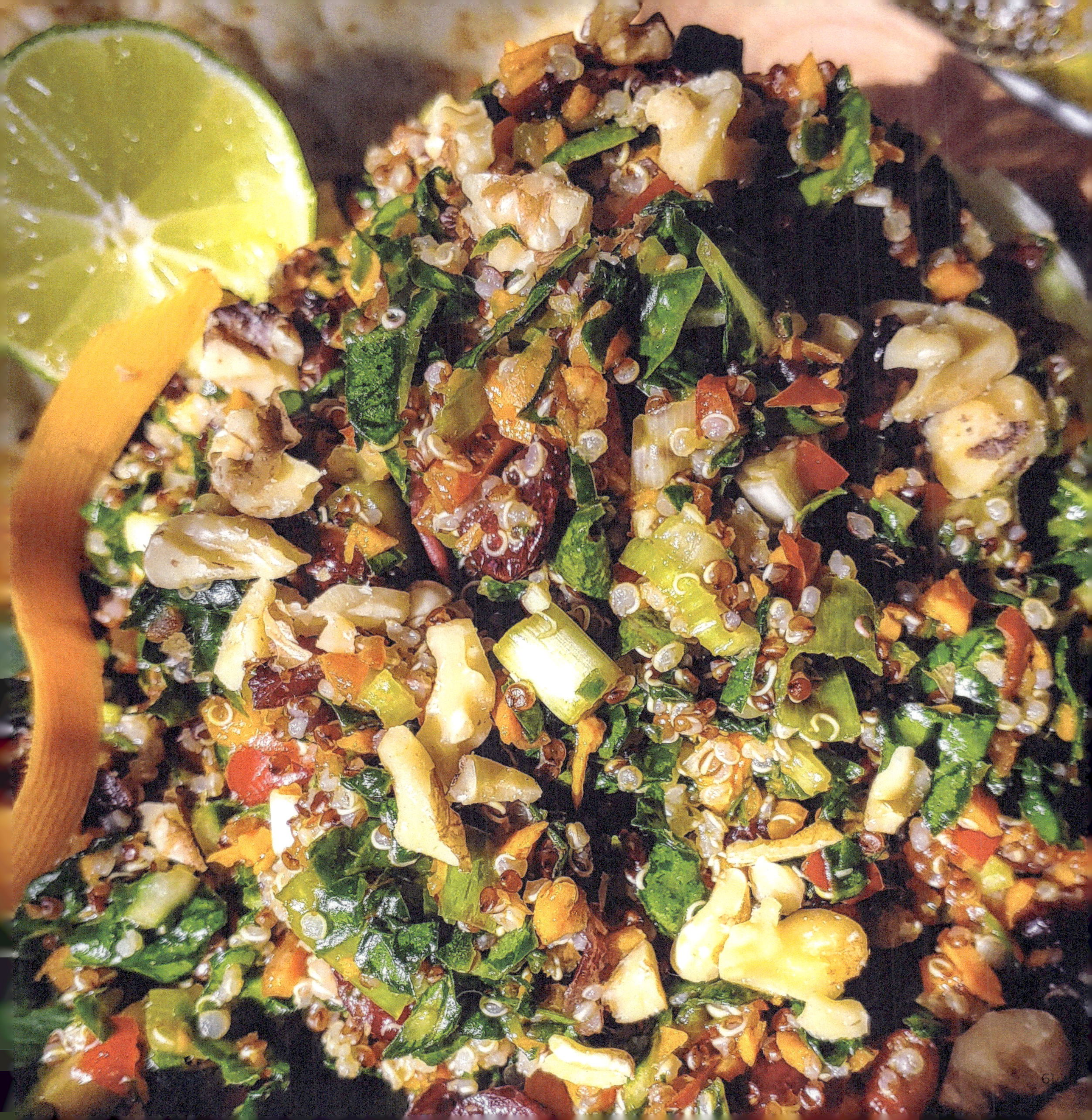

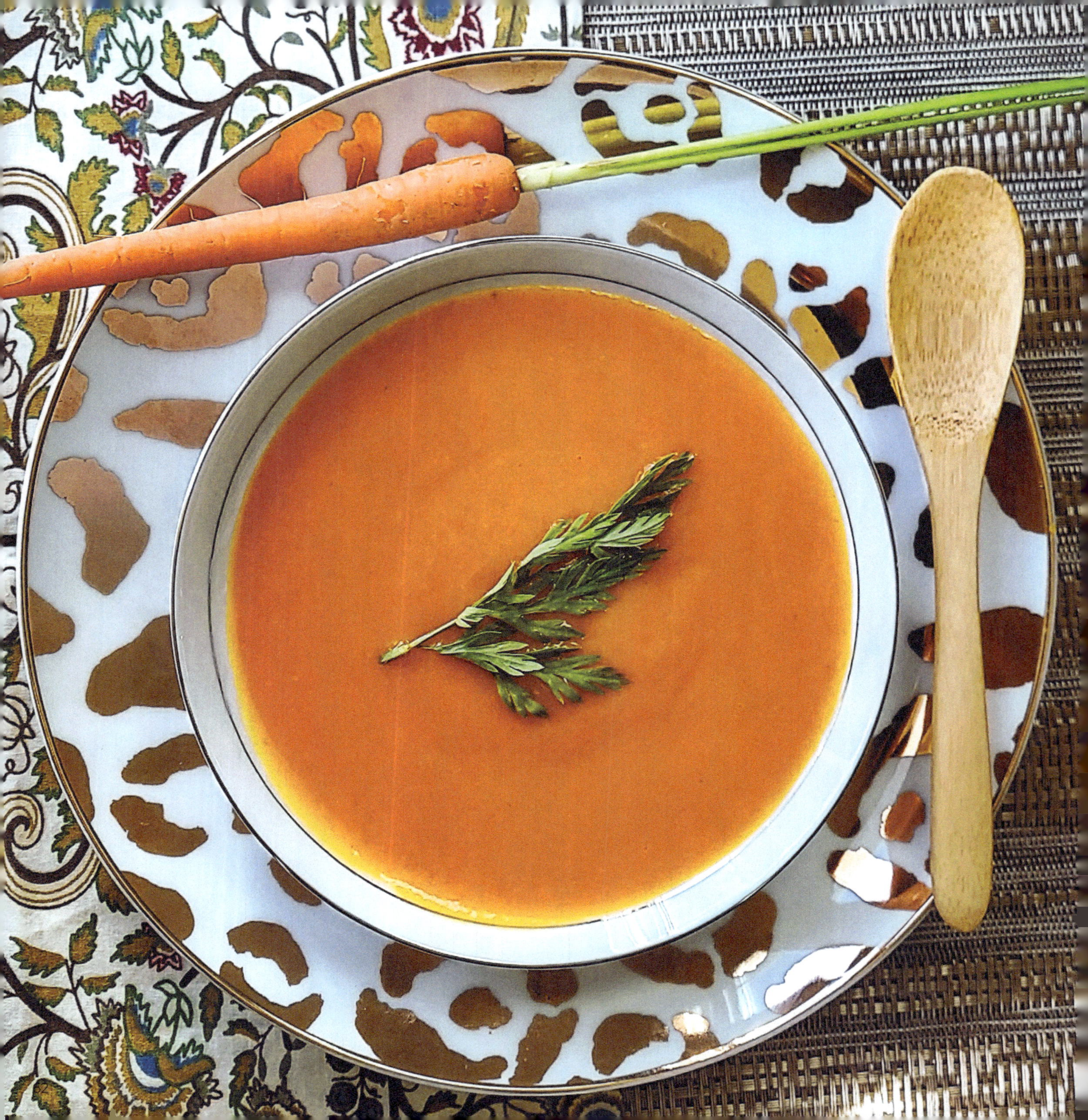

CARROT, TANGERINE, GINGER SOUP

Carrots, a root vegetable often used for flavoring, have the center stage in this recipe. The tangerine juice and freshly grated ginger fuels this soup! You can also drink this like a soothing tonic. Carrots are super high in fiber, vitamins, minerals, and antioxidants.

INGREDIENTS:

1 tablespoon coconut oil
½ cup sweet onion, chopped
1 rib celery, chopped
2 cloves garlic, chopped
3 cups vegetable stock (see recipe page. 135)
1½ pounds carrots (3 cups), chopped
3 pitted dates or 1 tablespoon raw honey
1 cup fresh tangerine juice
1 ½" piece ginger root, peeled and grated
½ teaspoon Celtic sea salt

PREPARATION:

1. In a large soup pot, warm coconut oil over medium-low heat. Add onions, celery, and garlic and sauté for 3 minutes.
2. Add vegetable stock, carrots, and 2 cups water. Cover and cook until carrots are tender when pierced with a knife (15 -20 minutes). Allow to cool.
3. Carefully pour vegetables and liquid into a blender or nutri-bullet, add dates/ honey, tangerine juice, grated ginger, and salt (if using). An immersion blender can also be used. Blend until smooth.

Makes 32 ounces

BOK CHOY WITH SOBA NOODLES

In this recipe Bok Choy, a crunchy Asia green is paired with soba noodles. Soba noodles are made from buckwheat, when not 100% buckwheat, they can also contain wheat. Soba is Japanese for buckwheat and these noodles are a non-gluten, nutritious alternative to pasta.

INGREDIENTS:

4 ounces soba noodles
1 teaspoon olive oil
3 cloves of garlic, diced
3 green onion, chopped
6 ounces button mushrooms, sliced
1 teaspoon of ground ginger
1 pound bok choy, chopped
2 teaspoons coconut aminos
1 teaspoon pepper; salt is optional
¼ cup of cilantro leaves, chopped
½ of small carrot, grated

PREPARATION:

1. Cook soba noodles first, following direction on package.
2. Bring 3 cups of water to a boil in a large pot. Add the soba noodles.
   Tip: Do not add salt to water. Use plenty of water so noodles do not sick.
   Do not over cook – or noodles may get mushy, 5-8 minutes only.
3. Rinse noodles well under cold water, drain in colander until ready to use.
4. Prepare Bok Choy - cut and remove the bottom and rinse each leaf, dry and cut into ribbons.
5. Warm olive oil in a skillet or wok over low heat. Add garlic and sauté for 2 minutes, Add onions and mushrooms and cover allowing to sweat for a minute or 2 until liquid builds. As liquid builds add the bok choy, sprinkle the ginger then add 2 cups of water. Increase the heat to medium-low and cook for 15 minutes.
6. Add the coconut aminos, and pepper. Add noodles to the skillet, toss to combine. Sprinkle the cilantro and carrots on top. Cover and cut off the heat.

Makes 4 servings

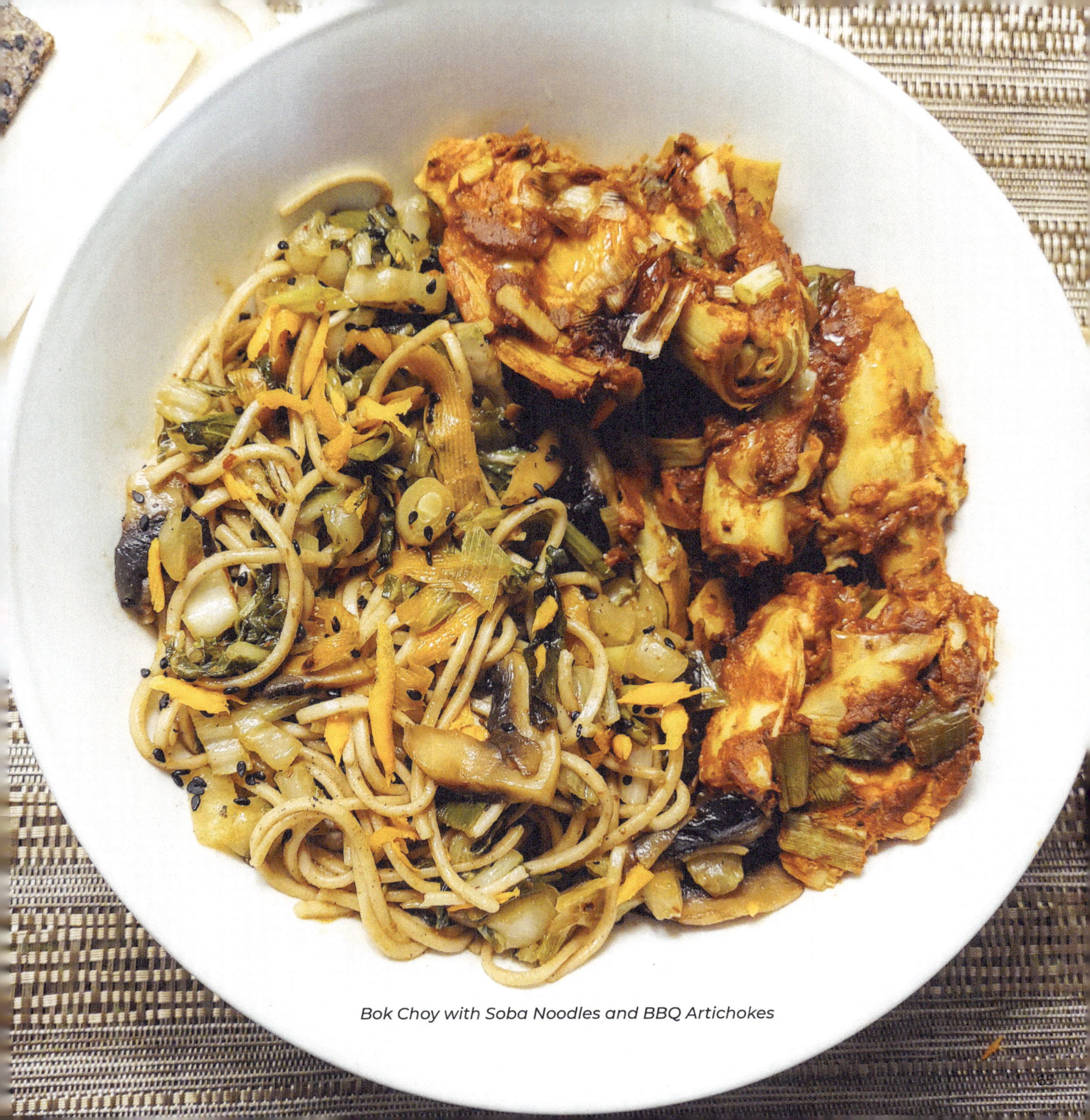

Bok Choy with Soba Noodles and BBQ Artichokes

BBQ ARTICHOKES

After enjoying roasted artichokes at a restaurant, I thought of this alternative dish with artichokes, and garlic and the barbecue sauce seem to work. Artichokes are a low-carb food, and are high in potassium.

INGREDIENTS:
2 cans/jars of artichoke hearts (approximately 9-12 artichokes)
2 cloves of garlic, sliced
1 cup BBQ sauce (see recipe page 200)
6 buns for serving: Optional

PREPARATION: Preheat oven to 375°F.

1. Pour artichoke hearts into colander, drain, rinse and pat dry. Slice artichoke hearts in half. Oil an oven-proof or cast iron pan with coconut oil. Place the artichokes in pan, add garlic slices, and ½ cup barbecue sauce to cover artichokes and place in pre-heated oven.
2. Bake for 30 minutes or until the artichokes are brown around the edges.
3. Serve roasted artichokes as a side or piled on a bun with remaining sauce.

Makes 4 to 6 servings

ASPARAGUS SPINACH ARUGULA SALAD

*Asparagus pairs well with spinach and arugula adds peppery delight.
These super greens are at their best in springtime and are high in antioxidants, including vitamin C and vitamin E.*

INGREDIENTS:
2 oranges, peel 1 orange, chop the segments
3 teaspoons whole-grain mustard (see page 196)
1 teaspoon flaxseed oil or olive oil
8-10 asparagus spears, ends trimmed, cut into 2" inch pieces
2 cups loosely packed spinach
2 cups loosely packed arugula
1 yellow bell pepper, sliced thinly

Prepare the ice water bath:
- Fill a bowl ½ full of ice
- Add water to fill ¾ of the bowl
- Blanch food in boiling water
- Transfer food to ice bath and completely immerse it, let it sit until the food is completely cold

DRESSING:
1. Juice from (1) orange
2. Make dressing: whisk together the orange juice, mustard, and oil.

PREPARATION:

1. Prepare a bowl of ice and water for the ice bath (see inset).
2. In a large pot over high heat, bring 3 cups of water to a boil.
3. Immerse the asparagus in the boiling water, cover, and blanch for 3 minutes.
4. Use a slotted spoon to move asparagus to the ice-water to stop it from cooking any further. (This will keep the asparagus crisp and retain its bright color). Drain and set aside.
5. Arrange spinach and arugula in bowls. Add asparagus, bell pepper, and orange segments. Serve with this light dressing.

Makes 4 servings

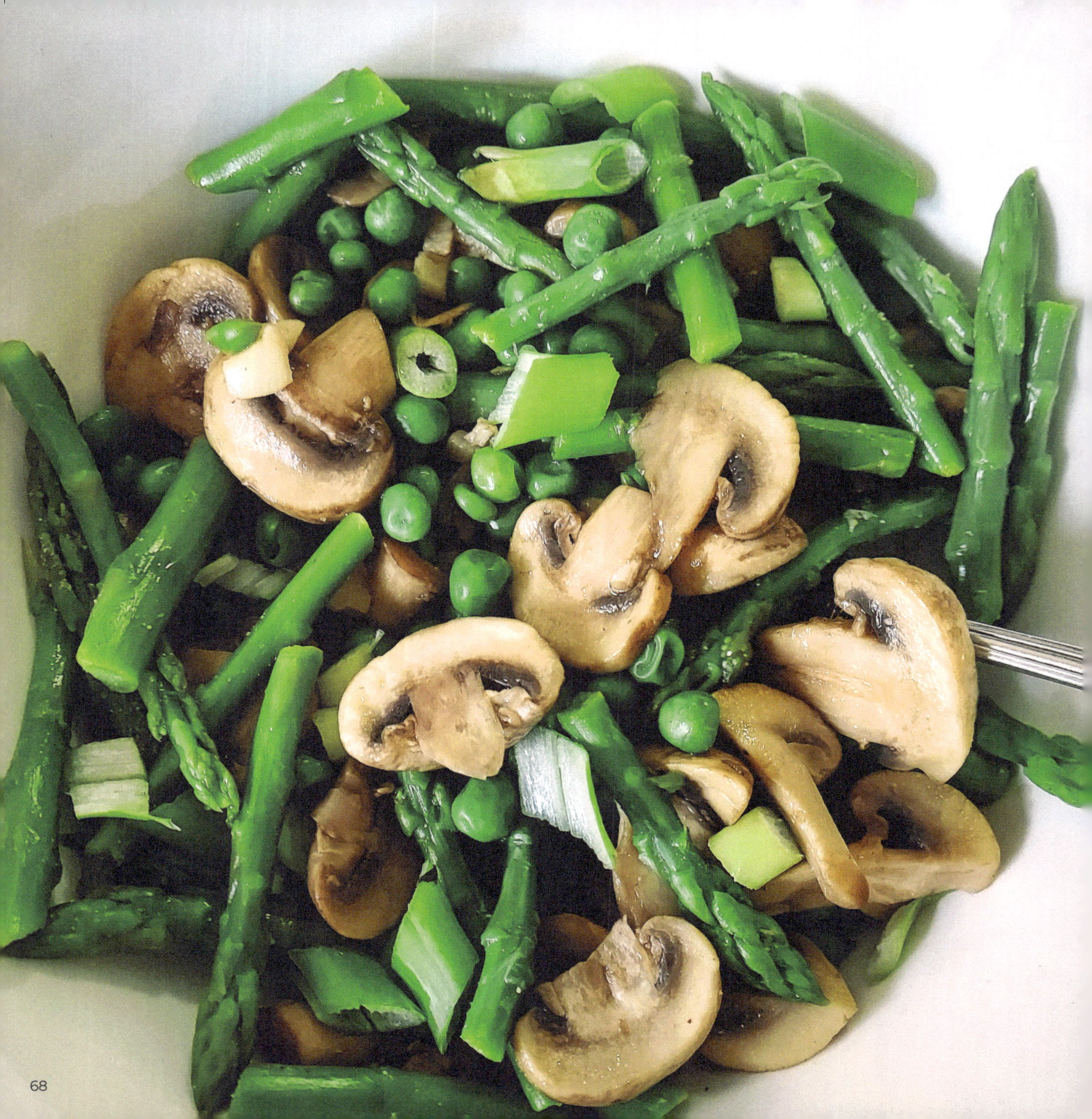

SPRING VEGETABLE BOWL

The sweetness of the spring peas, asparagus, and mushrooms make a simple, delicious, and healthy vegetable bowl.

INGREDIENTS:

15 asparagus spears, trimmed and cut diagonally into 2" pieces
1 teaspoon olive oil
One 8-ounce package of mushrooms (button or cremini) sliced
1 clove garlic, minced
One 12-ounce bag frozen spring peas
3 green onions, cut 1/8 in thick

DRESSING:

Juice of 2 oranges
Juice of 1 lime
1 -2 teaspoons whole grain mustard
¼ teaspoon onion powder
Celtic sea salt and pepper to taste

PREPARATION:

1. In a large saucepan, bring 3 cups of water to a boil. Add asparagus and blanch for 3 minutes. Move asparagus to an ice water bath (see page 67). Once the asparagus stalks are cold (i.e., the cooking process has stopped), remove them from the ice water with a slotted spoon and drain.

2. Warm olive oil in a medium-size skillet over low heat. Add mushrooms and garlic and cover. Allow mushrooms to sweat for 1-2 minutes. Uncover and cook until liquid is absorbed. Add frozen peas and cook for approximately 2 minutes. Drain mushrooms and peas through a strainer.

3. Transfer the drained mushrooms and peas to a bowl. Mix in the asparagus and green onions. Serve with dressing.

Makes 4 servings

CHICKPEA TUNA

This dish is one of my granddaughter Kennedy's favorite—as a toddler, she loved the avocado replacing the mayonnaise. You may prefer to use mayonnaise or salad dressing.

INGREDIENTS:

2 cups cooked chickpeas or one 15-ounce can of chickpeas
½ of a medium onion, diced
1 rib celery, diced
1-2 tablespoons sweet relish
½ avocado, peeled and mash

PREPARATION:

1. For can chickpeas - drain and rinse them thoroughly. Place the chickpeas in a bowl and mash with a fork or in small chopper. Add the onion, celery, and relish. mix well.

2. Blend mashed avocado into the chickpeas.

Makes 4 servings

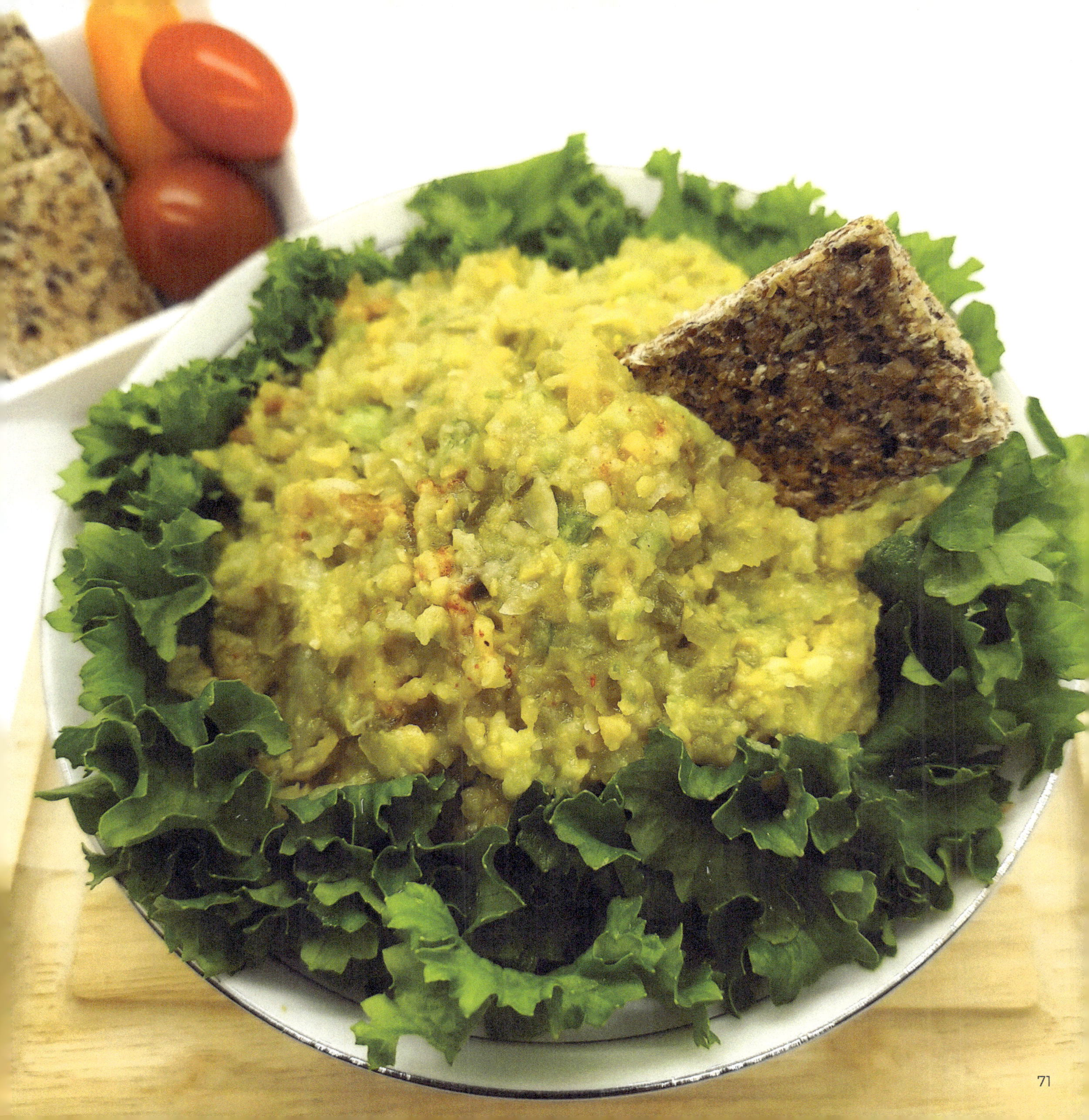

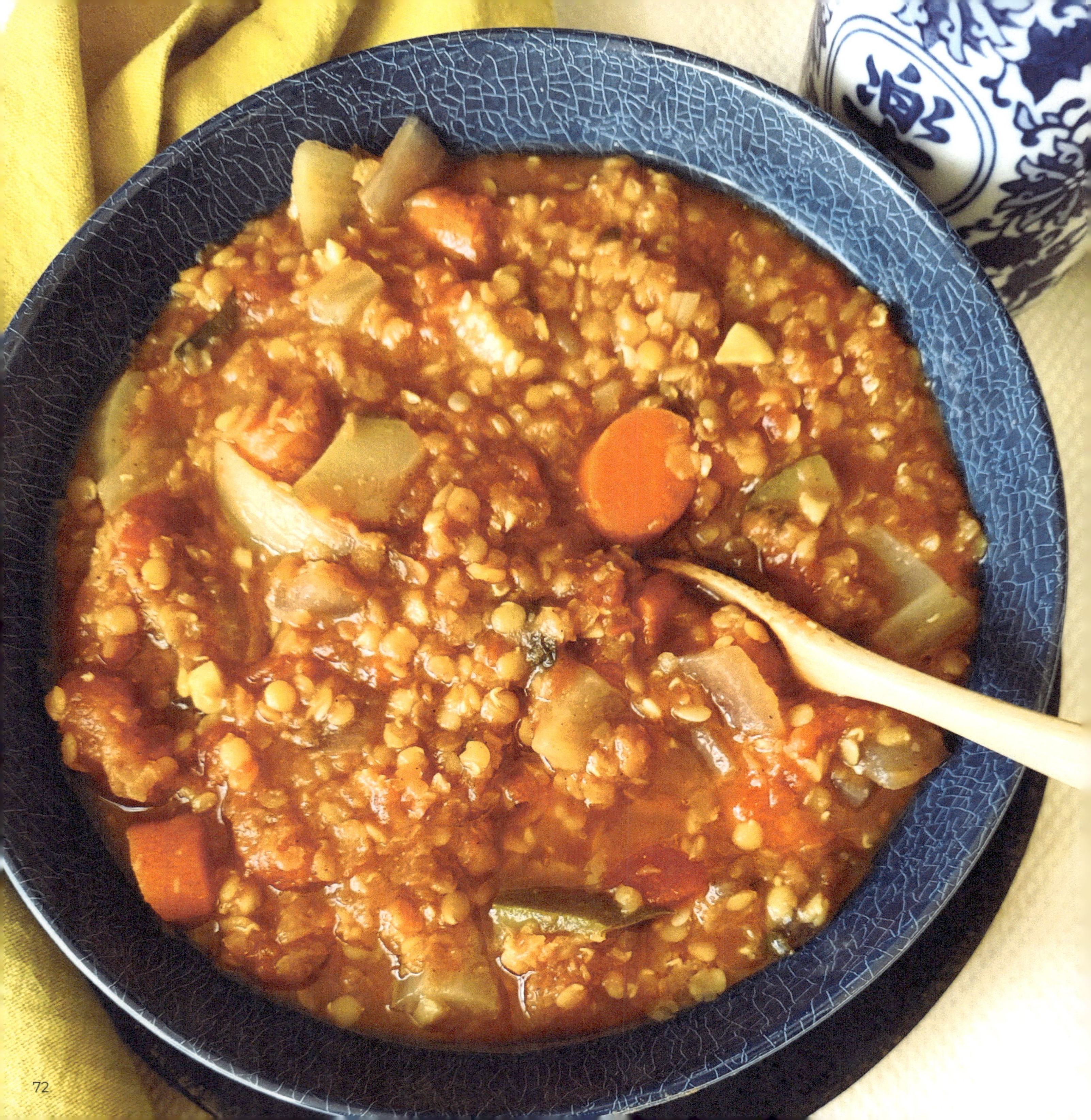

RED LENTIL SOUP

This lentil dish is included with the spring dishes because it features fennel. A fresh fennel bulb adds a crunchy texture and just enough flavor to be noticed. Lentils transcend all seasons; they are an excellent source of dietary fiber, copper, phosphorus, and manganese. They are also sources of protein, iron, zinc, potassium, Vitamin B1, and vitamin B6.

INGREDIENTS:

3 cups of vegetable broth or water, divided
1 small red onion, chopped (1/2 cup)
1 fennel bulb, chopped
3 cloves garlic, diced
2 carrots, chopped
1 teaspoon ground ginger
1 teaspoon curry powder
1 teaspoon ground chili
One 28-ounce can of roma tomatoes with juice, chopped
3/4 cup dry red lentils, rinsed well
2 bay leaves
½ teaspoon celtic sea salt
1 small zucchini, chopped

PREPARATION:

1. 3/4 cup dry red lentils, rinse until water is clear and set aside.
2. In a large soup pot over low heat. Add ½ cup of the water or vegetable broth, onion and fennel and sauté for 2 minutes, add garlic and cook 2 minutes.
3. Add carrots and spices and stir well. Add tomatoes with juice, lentils, the remaining water or vegetable broth and bay leaves. Increase heat bring everything to a medium boil, then reduce heat to low simmer, cook for 10 minutes.
4. Add zucchini, sprinkle in sea salt. Add water or broth if too thick cook 15 minutes or until the zucchini is translucent. Remove bay leaves before serving.

Makes 4 servings

Summer Vegetables and Fruits
(partial listing)

Bell Peppers
Cucumbers
Eggplant
Green Beans
Okra
Onions
Summer Squash
Tomatoes
Zucchini

Apricots
Blackberries
Blueberries
Cantaloup
Cherries
Nectarines
Peaches
Plums
Strawberries
Watermelon

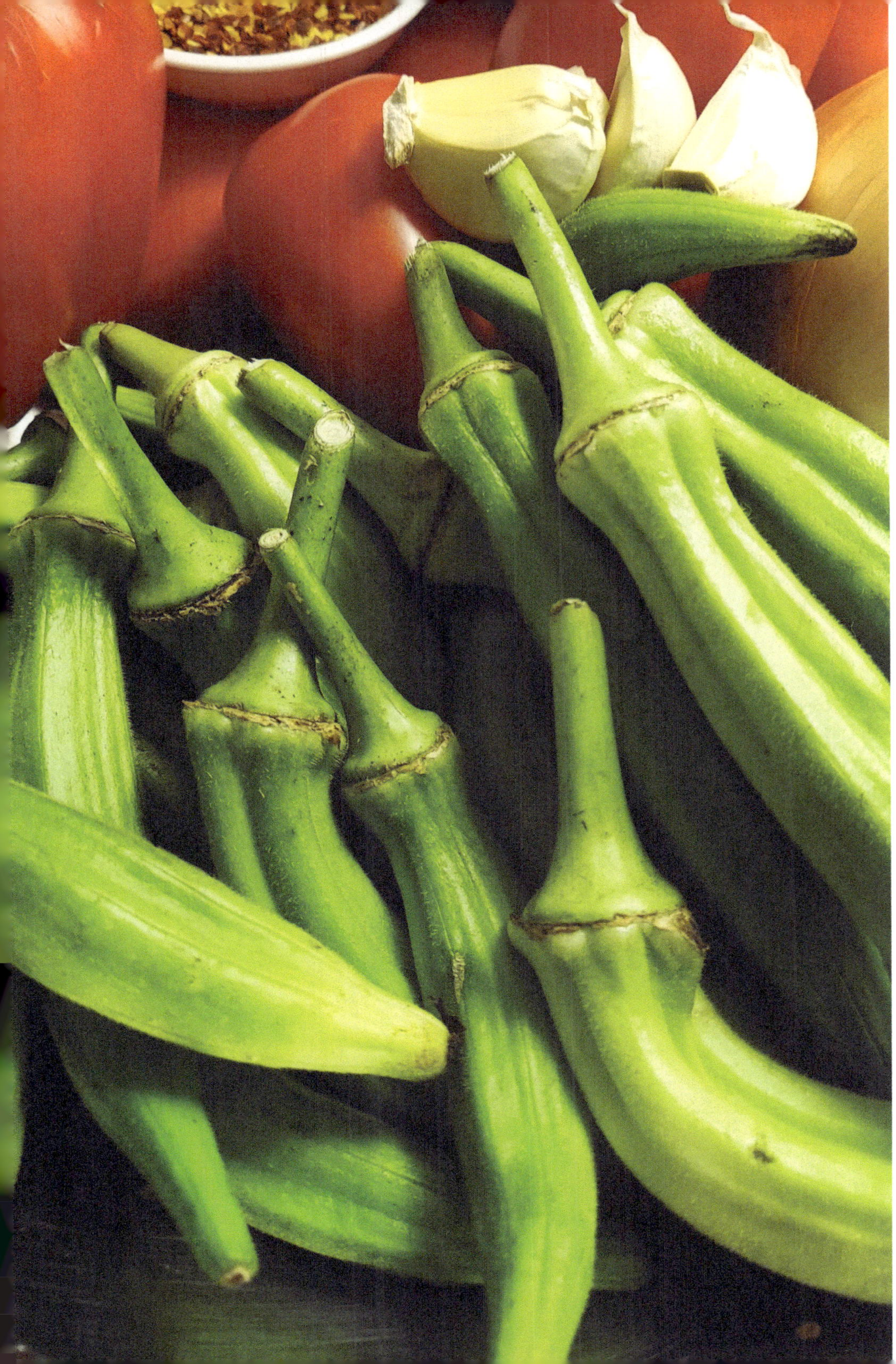

SUMMER

JUNE, JULY + AUGUST

SUMMER RECIPES

Summer has arrived! Warm mornings turn into hot days, short days are lengthened so the sun sets well into the evening. A season to enjoy warm weather and luscious, summer fruits including: cantaloupe, honeydew, casaba melon, plums, peaches, nectarines, watermelon, Asian pears, apricots, figs, jackfruit, and key limes. These fruits can be eaten alone or combined in an unlimited number of ways: raw in salads, cooked into fruit pies and tarts, or blended into refreshing summer smoothies.

We have our summer vegetables: green okra, lima beans, bell peppers, corn, eggplant, zucchini, garlic, Chinese long beans, and a variety of summer squash. These wonderful vegetables are to be grilled, sautéed, roasted, made into cold or warm soups, used raw in salads, or grated into slaws. We cannot forget the all-time summer favorites: tomatoes and cucumbers.

Eating seasonally means rotating food with the season. It's an exciting lifestyle choice! Seasonal vegetables and fruits can also be preserved to enjoy into the next seasons. It's so awesome to enjoy Summer strawberries you preserved in the summer months in your strawberry jam during the Christmas holiday. Or to include Roma tomatoes you preserved from the summer months in your winter stews, soups, and sauces.

Most summer fruits and vegetables are cooling foods, which is to say, these foods help the body stay cool and refreshed. Using certain spices through the summer months can also add a cooling effect, as they can help you cool down through sweating.

Let's welcome summer!

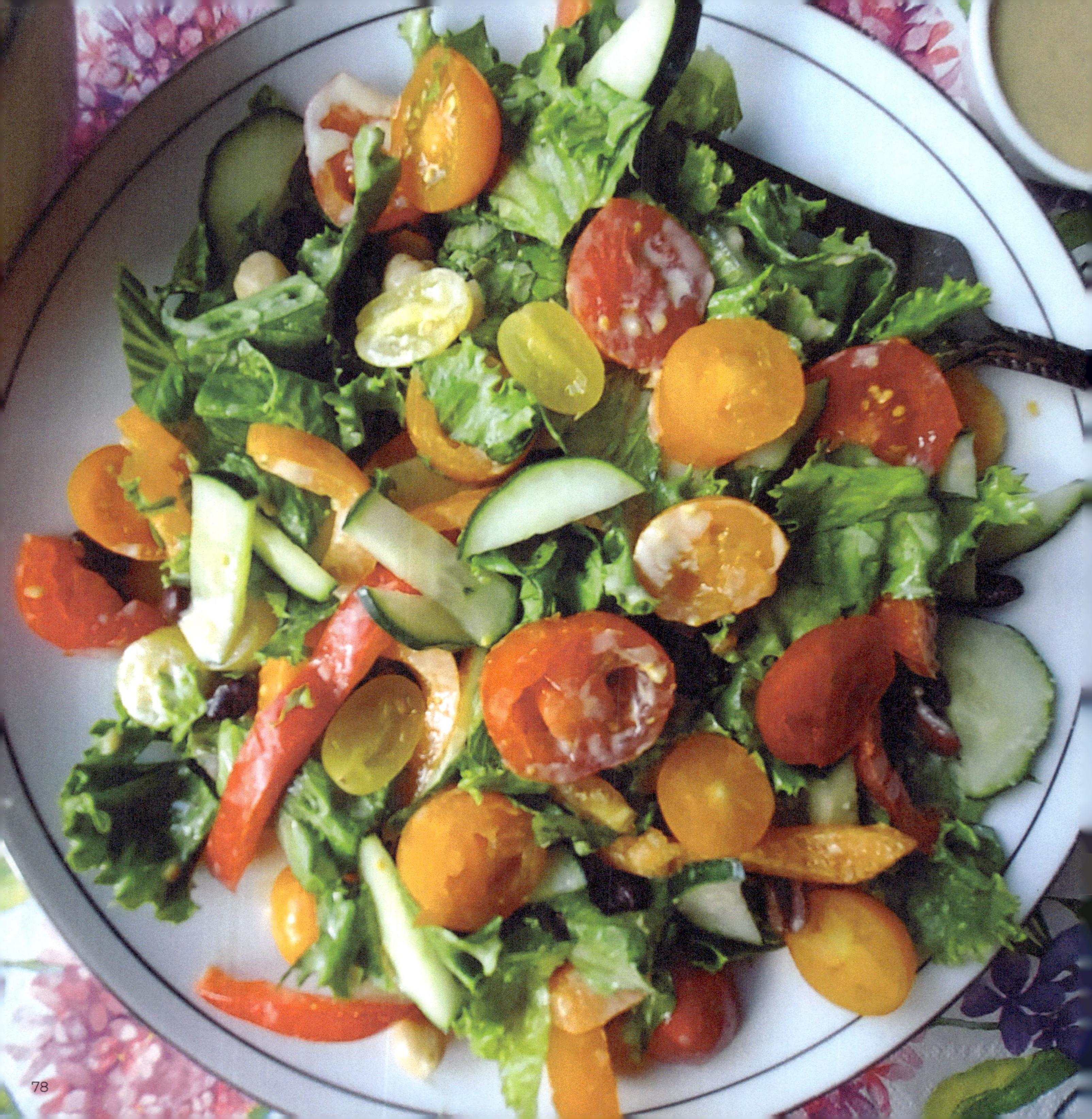

SUMMER VEGGIE POWER SALAD

Enjoy this bowl of delicious summer veggies popping with color and rich in vitamins, minerals, and nutrients. Let's toss it up, dig in, and enjoy the sunshine! Beans are included as a protein source, and the cucumbers are a food source of electrolytes like magnesium, sodium, phosphorus, and calcium. Top with luscious tahini-lime dressing.

INGREDIENTS:

4-6 cups lettuce (any variety), rinsed and dried
1 red bell pepper, diced
1 yellow bell pepper, diced
1 cup cherry tomatoes, halved
1 cup cooked (or canned) chickpeas
1 English or regular cucumber, sliced thinly
4 green onions, sliced
Optional: Avocado, sliced
Tahini-Lime dressing for serving (see page 199)

PREPARATION:

1. Place the greens in large salad bowl or platter and add the remaining ingredients. Toss well to combine. Serve with dressing.

Makes 4 to 6 servings

CABBAGE & PURPLE KOHLRABI SLAW

The beautiful purple color and flawless green leaves of the kohlrabi were what intrigued me to purchase it for the first time. Kohlrabi is a member of the cabbage family and is a great source of vitamin C, vitamin B, iron, potassium, calcium, phosphorus, copper, and iron. The leaves are large, like collards. The flavor of a kohlrabi bulb is mild, and is a wonderful vegetable to work with—it's pliable, not stiff. It's great for slaw!

INGREDIENTS:

¼ head small red cabbage, thinly sliced
¼ head small Savoy cabbage, thinly sliced
2-3 kohlrabi leaves, rolled into cylinders and slice thin
¼ small red onion, sliced thin
1 clove garlic, diced
½ purple kohlrabi bulb, peeled and grated
2 tablespoons tahini
1 teaspoon apple cider vinegar
1 teaspoon whole-grain mustard *(see page 196)*
1 tablespoon maple syrup
1 teaspoon fresh lime juice
Celtic sea salt and pepper to taste
Sesame Seed Sprinkles - Optional

PREPARATION:

1. In a large salad bowl, place the red and savoy cabbage, kohlrabi leaves, onion, garlic, and the grated kohlrabi bulb.

2. In a small bowl, whisk together the tahini, vinegar, mustard, maple syrup, 2 tablespoons of water, lime juice, salt and pepper to taste. Drizzle the dressing over the slaw and mix well. Sesame seed sprinkles as an option.

Makes 4 servings

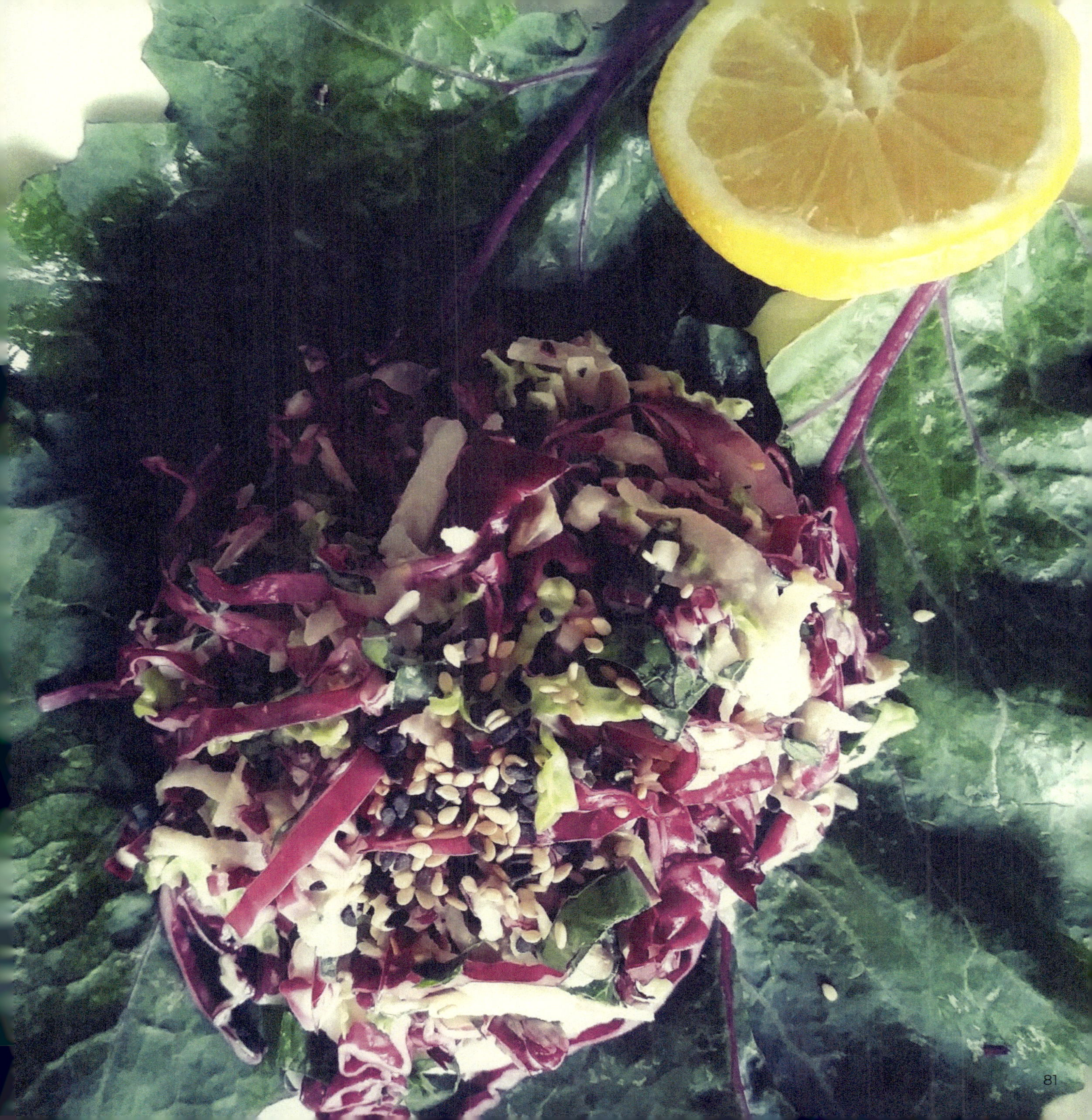

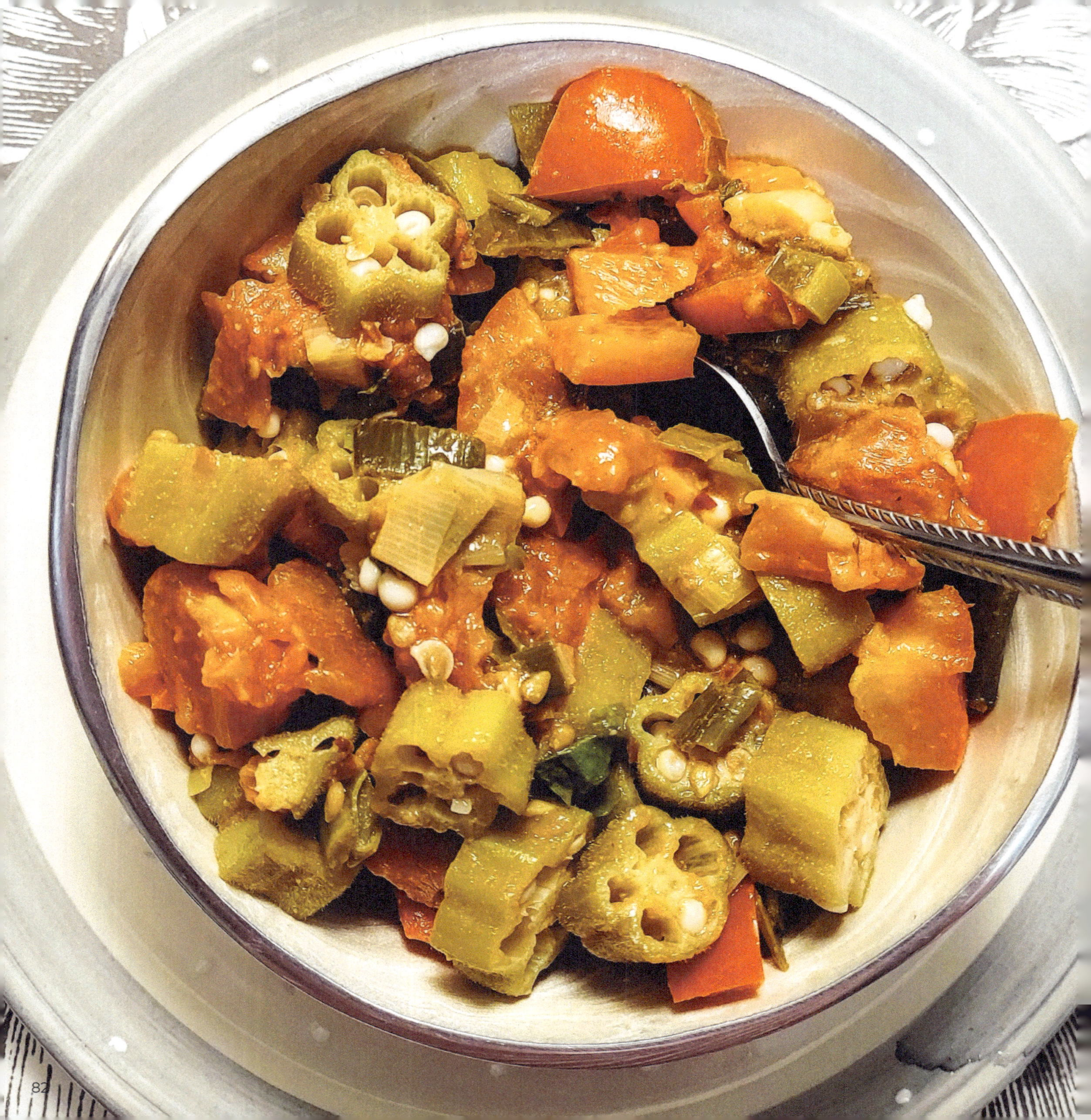

CORN, OKRA & TOMATOES...HOLD THE CORN

Fresh okra is most abundant during the summer. It is a great source of fiber, vitamin B6, and folate, and has recently been suggested to support blood sugar maintenance. Cooking the okra fast instead of a slow simmer reduced the viscosity usually associated with okra.

INGREDIENTS:

1 tablespoon olive oil
1 medium onion, chopped (1 cup)
3 cloves garlic, minced
5 roma tomatoes, chopped (2-1/2 cups)
½ fresh red bell pepper, diced
1 teaspoon onion powder
1½ teaspoon ground cumin
¼ teaspoon red pepper flakes
2 cups fresh okra, cut into ¼" inch-thick slices
½ teaspoon Celtic sea salt
Cooked rice for serving

PREPARATION:

1. Warm olive oil in a medium-size saucepan over medium-low heat. Add onions and sauté for 2 minutes, then add garlic and cook for 1 additional minute.
2. Stir in tomatoes and red bell peppers and cook for 5 minutes. Add 1 cup of water and stir in the, onion powder, cumin, and red pepper flakes. Add okra, Celtic sea salt and reduce/lower heat to low.
3. Cook 15-20 minutes, stirring occasionally, add water if needed. Cook until okra is tender. (Add more water if needed.) Can be served over rice or alone as a side.

Makes 4 to 6 servings

CHICKPEA-BEET NUGGETS

Garbanzo beans (also known as chickpeas) make delicious, healthy veggie burgers. The beans are high in protein, low in fat and sodium, and are packed with beneficial nutrients. I made the mixture into small nuggets and, served them with handcrafted sauce, which was a great hit.

INGREDIENTS:

1 tablespoon ground flaxseeds
1 teaspoon olive oil
1 small onion, diced
2 cloves garlic, minced
1 teaspoon dried thyme
1 teaspoon ground cumin
1 teaspoon smoked paprika
½ of a small beet, grated
¼ teaspoon Celtic sea salt
1 ½ cups cooked chickpeas or one 15-ounce can chickpeas, rinsed and mashed
½ cup walnuts, finely ground

PREPARATION: Preheat oven to 375°F.

1. In a small bowl, mix ground flaxseeds with 3 tablespoons water. Let the mixture stand for 3 minutes to thicken.

2. Add oil and onion to a medium-size skillet over low heat. Stir in garlic and cook for 3 minutes. Add thyme, spices, beets, and salt. Cover and turn the heat off.

3. In a medium mixing bowl, add the mashed chickpeas, cooked vegetables, flaxseed mixture, and ground walnuts. Mix well. If the mixture is too moist to easily form into patties, add additional ground walnuts as needed.

4. Form the mixture into small nuggets or large patties and place them on a baking sheet lined with parchment paper. Bake for 15 minutes on each side.

Makes 12 nuggets or 4 patties

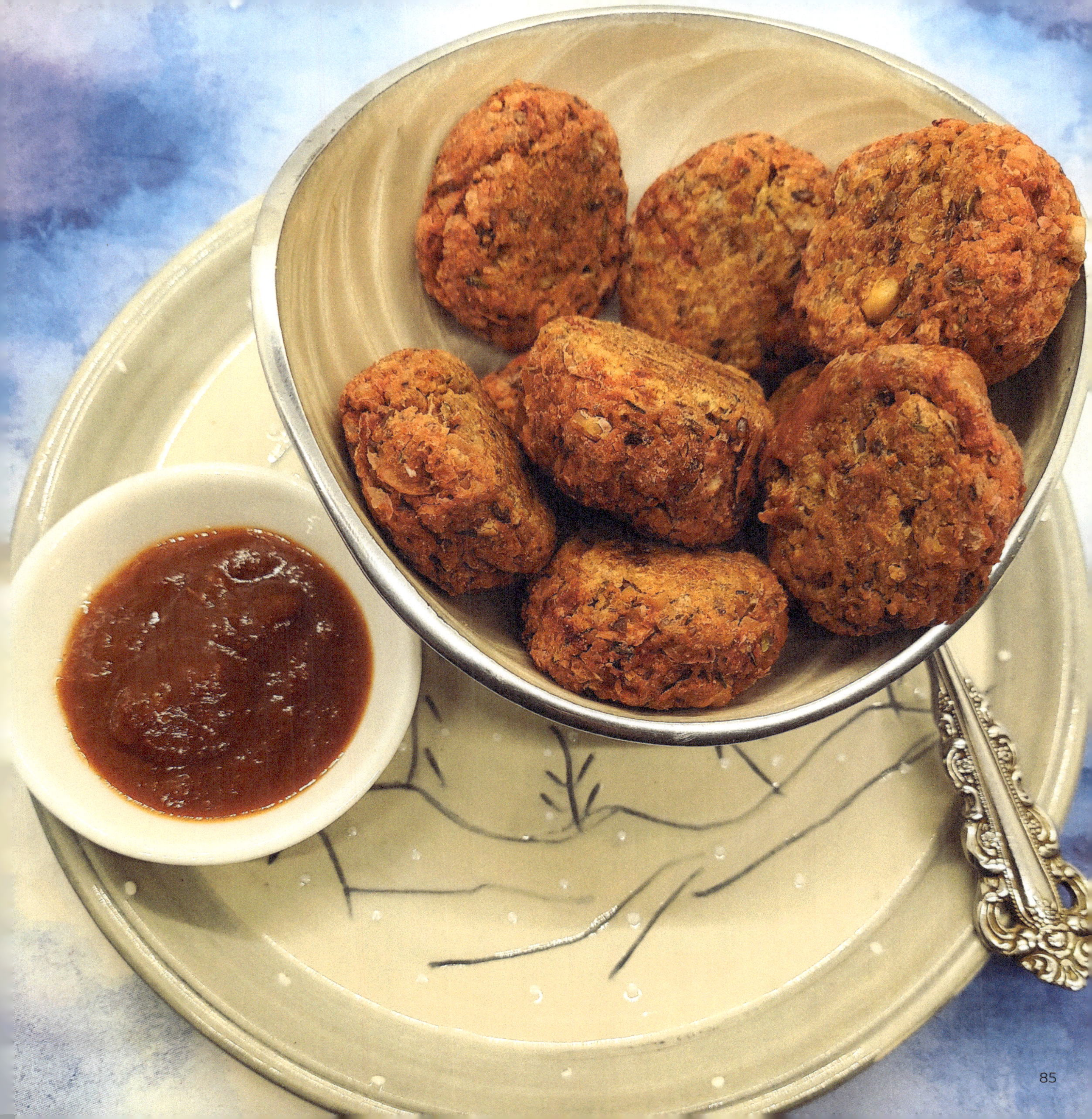

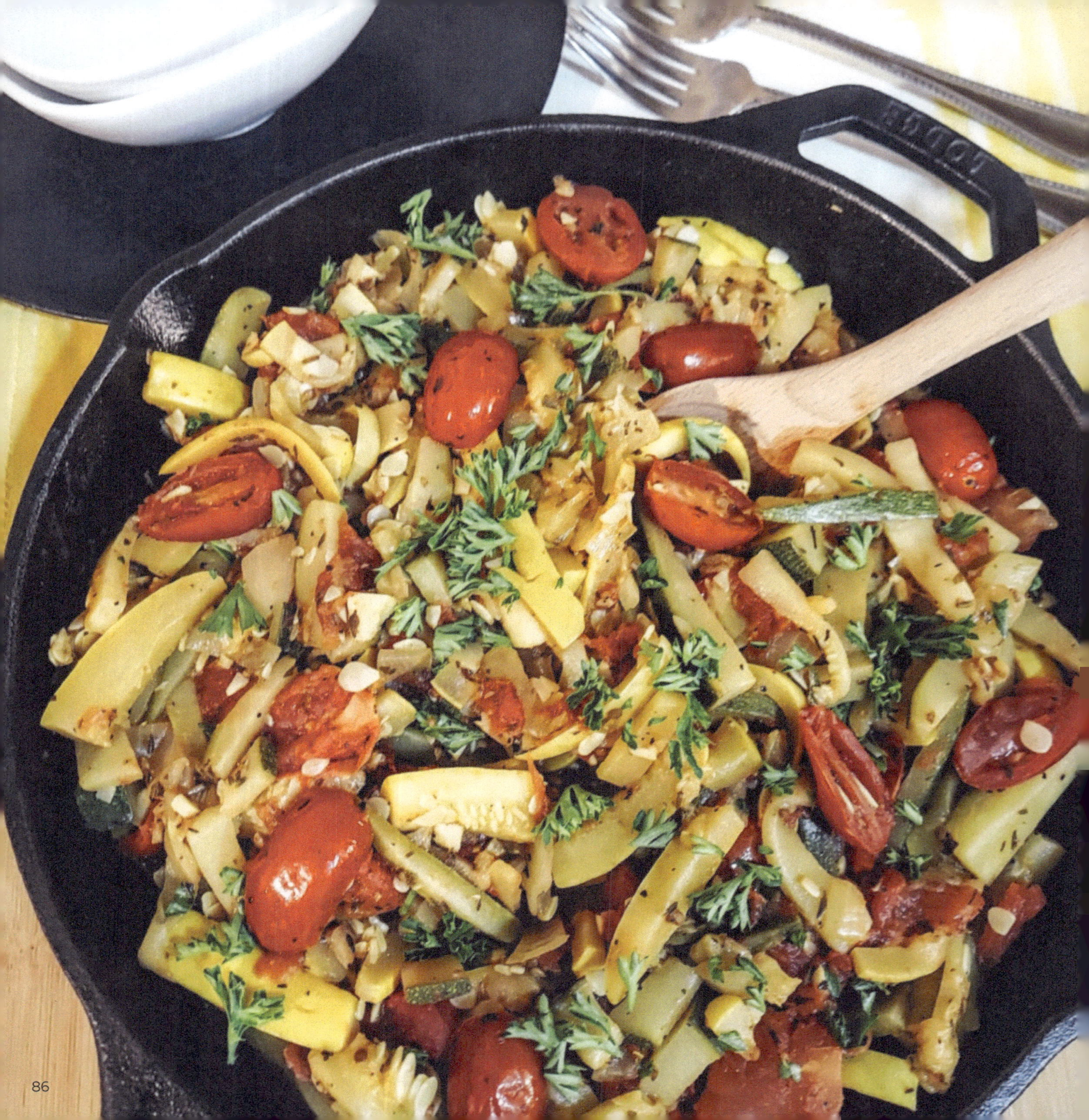
LODGE

ZUCCHINI, TOMATO & SQUASH MEDLEY

Summer gardens usually have an overabundance of squash. Here is a dish that uses a medley of seasonal zucchini, summer squash, and tomatoes.

INGREDIENTS:

1 tablespoon olive oil
1 medium onion, chopped
3 cloves garlic, minced
6 plum, tomatoes, cut into quarters
1 pint cherry tomatoes, cut into halves
2 teaspoons fresh lemon juice
1 teaspoon dried oregano
1 teaspoon dried thyme
1 teaspoon ground turmeric
1 teaspoon ground ginger
½ teaspoon Celtic sea salt
Dash of cayenne pepper
1 large zucchini squash, cut into matchsticks*
2 medium yellow crookneck squash, cut into matchsticks*
Handful flat-leaf parsley, chopped

Matchstick cut:
Cut off both ends of squash. Cut crosswise into equal segments and cut segments into 2" sections. Slice sections lengthwise into stabs. Stack stabs, then slice into 8"-long sticks.

Optional: Cooked rice or noodles for serving.

PREPARATION:

1. Warm olive oil in a large skillet over medium-low heat. Add onion and sauté for 2 minutes, then add the garlic and stir continuously for 1 minute as it cooks..
2. Add tomatoes and cook for 5-6 minutes, mash them with the back of a spoon to release their juice. Stir in ½ cup of water.
3. Add lemon juice, herbs, spices, salt, and pepper and blend well. Stir in the squash. Simmer over low heat for 20 minutes or until the vegetables are soft and the liquid is fragrant. Sprinkle in the parsley.
4. May be served over rice or noodles.

Makes 4 to 6 servings

CURRIED QUINOA

This curried quinoa dish can be made with any variation of quinoa: red, black, or tan. Cooking a large batch of quinoa works well as you will then have this extremely nutritious and very versatile grain on hand to use in a variety of ways.

INGREDIENTS:

1 cup dry quinoa, rinsed thoroughly
½ yellow onion, diced
1 teaspoon ground turmeric
1 teaspoon ground ginger
1 teaspoon ground coriander
1 teaspoon ground cinnamon

PREPARATION:

1. Add the rinsed quinoa and 2 cups of water to a medium pot, over medium heat. Stir in the spices, cover and bring to a boil.

2. Once boiling, reduce heat to low and simmer covered for 15 minutes or until the quinoa has absorbed the cooking liquid. Allow to cool and fluff with a fork.

Makes 4 to 6 servings

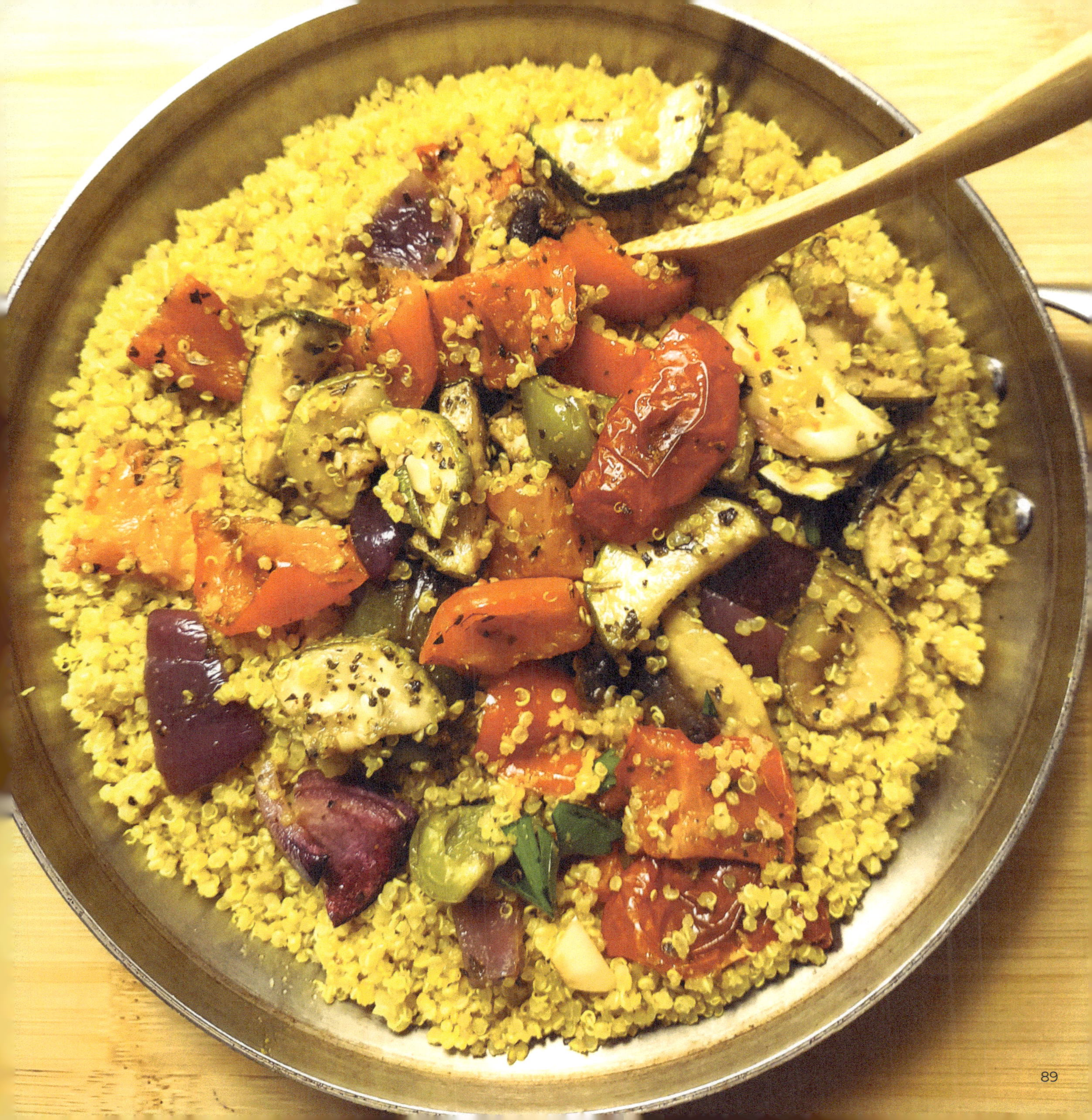

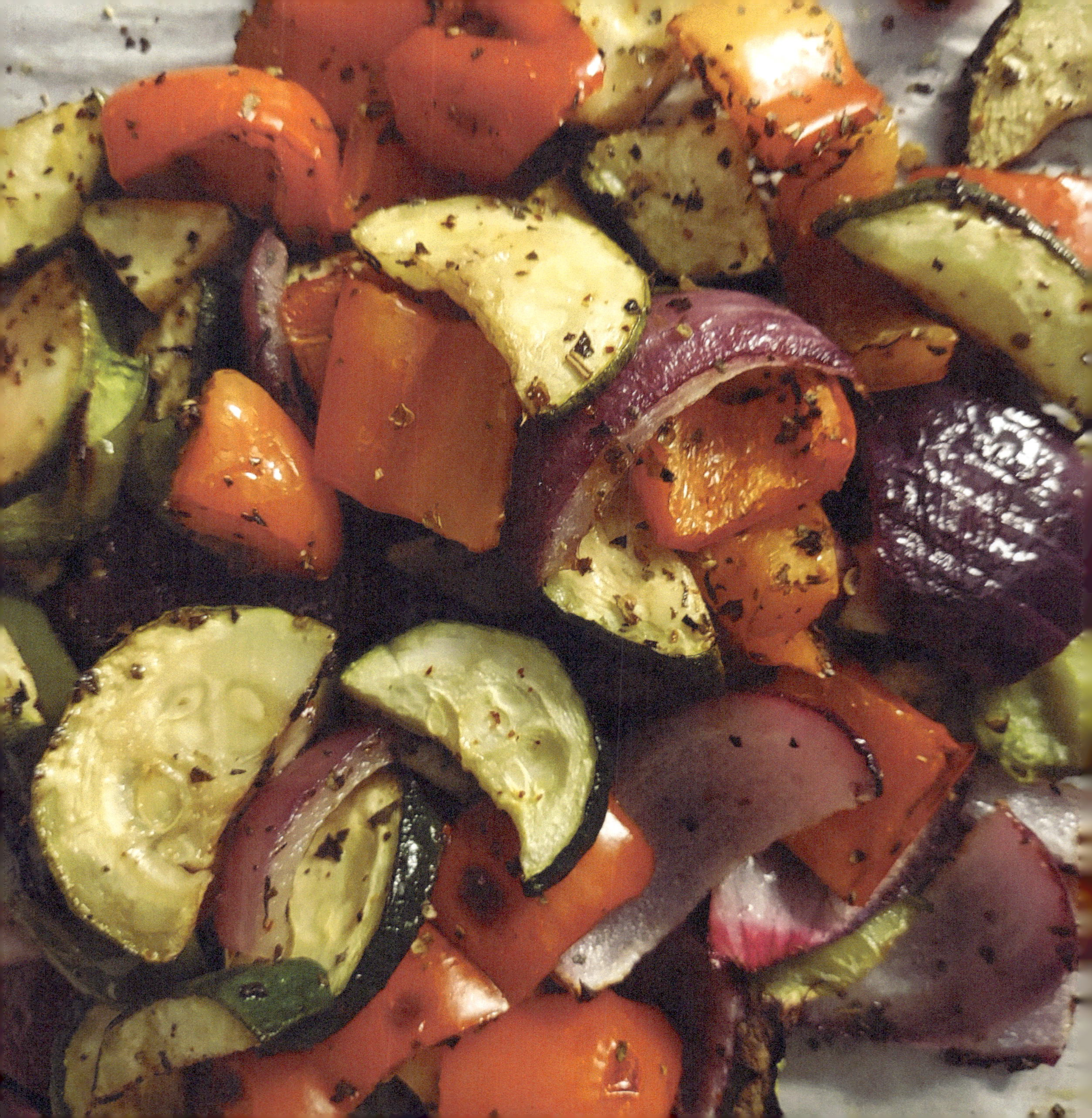

ROASTED/GRILLED VEGGIES

Roasting brings out the natural sweetness in most vegetables. Feel free to use your choice of vegetables when roasting! It's best to cut veggies into uniform sizes so they cook evenly. The vegetables in this recipe have the same cooking time. Always remember to roast vegetables according to their cook time. Root vegetables may take 25 to 40 minutes, cruciferous vegetables roast in 20 to 30 minutes, soft vegetables roast in 10 to 20 minutes. Give veggies room to roast—if not, they will steam.

INGREDIENTS:

1 red onion, quartered
1 red bell pepper, cut into 1" strips
1 green bell pepper, cut into 1" strips
1 zucchini, sliced into rounds
1 summer squash, sliced into rounds
1 cup button or baby portabella (also called cremini) mushrooms, halved or sliced
2 Roma tomatoes, quartered
½ teaspoon dried basil
1 teaspoon olive oil
½ tablespoon balsamic vinegar
Celtic sea salt and pepper to taste
For Serving: Curried Quinoa (see page 88)
Flaxseed oil for drizzling

PREPARATION: Preheat oven to 425°F.

1. Place all ingredients except for the quinoa and flaxseed oil in a large bowl. Toss the vegetables by hand to ensure that they are well-coated.
2. Arrange vegetables on a parchment-lined baking sheet and roast for 25 minutes or until evenly browned. (Check them occasionally and given a quick stir!).
3. The veggies can be served over curried quinoa with a drizzle of flaxseed oil.

Makes 4 servings

BLACK BEAN-QUINOA BURGER

Black bean burgers are frequently the first veggie burger many people are introduced to. The ingredients are easily accessible and the burgers are tasty and quick to prepare. Black beans are high in plant protein, vitamins, and fiber. Quinoa is a soft, highly nutritious balance to the beans.

INGREDIENTS:

½ cup of dry red quinoa (or white) rinsed well
1 tablespoon olive oil
1 small onion, diced (1/2 cup)
2 cloves garlic, minced
1 teaspoon chili powder
1 teaspoon smoked paprika
1/2 teaspoon onion powder
1 teaspoon dried thyme
¼ teaspoon black pepper
A pinch of Celtic sea salt
One (15-ounce) can black beans, drain and rinse
1/2 cup rolled oats, ground into flour
4 buns or rolls

PREPARATION: Preheat oven to 375°F.

1. Combine quinoa and 1 cup of water in a saucepan over medium- high heat. Bring to a boil, reduce heat to simmer, cover and cook until all the water is absorbed. Fluff quinoa with a fork. Re-cover until ready to use.

2. Warm oil in a small skillet over low heat. Add the onions and garlic and sauté for 2 minutes. Stir in spices, thyme, pepper and salt. Turn off the heat and cover.

3. Place black beans in a bowl, with a fork mash them into a chunky mash. Add the onion mixture and quinoa to the bowl and blend well. Taste, adjust seasonings as needed.

4. Add ground oats a little at a time to firm the mixture. Knead the mixture. Let it set for up to 10 minutes before forming into patties (½ cup each). Place the patties on a baking sheet lined with parchment paper. Bake for 15 minutes on each side, remove from the oven, cool and enjoy on a bun with condiments of our choice.

Makes 6 patties

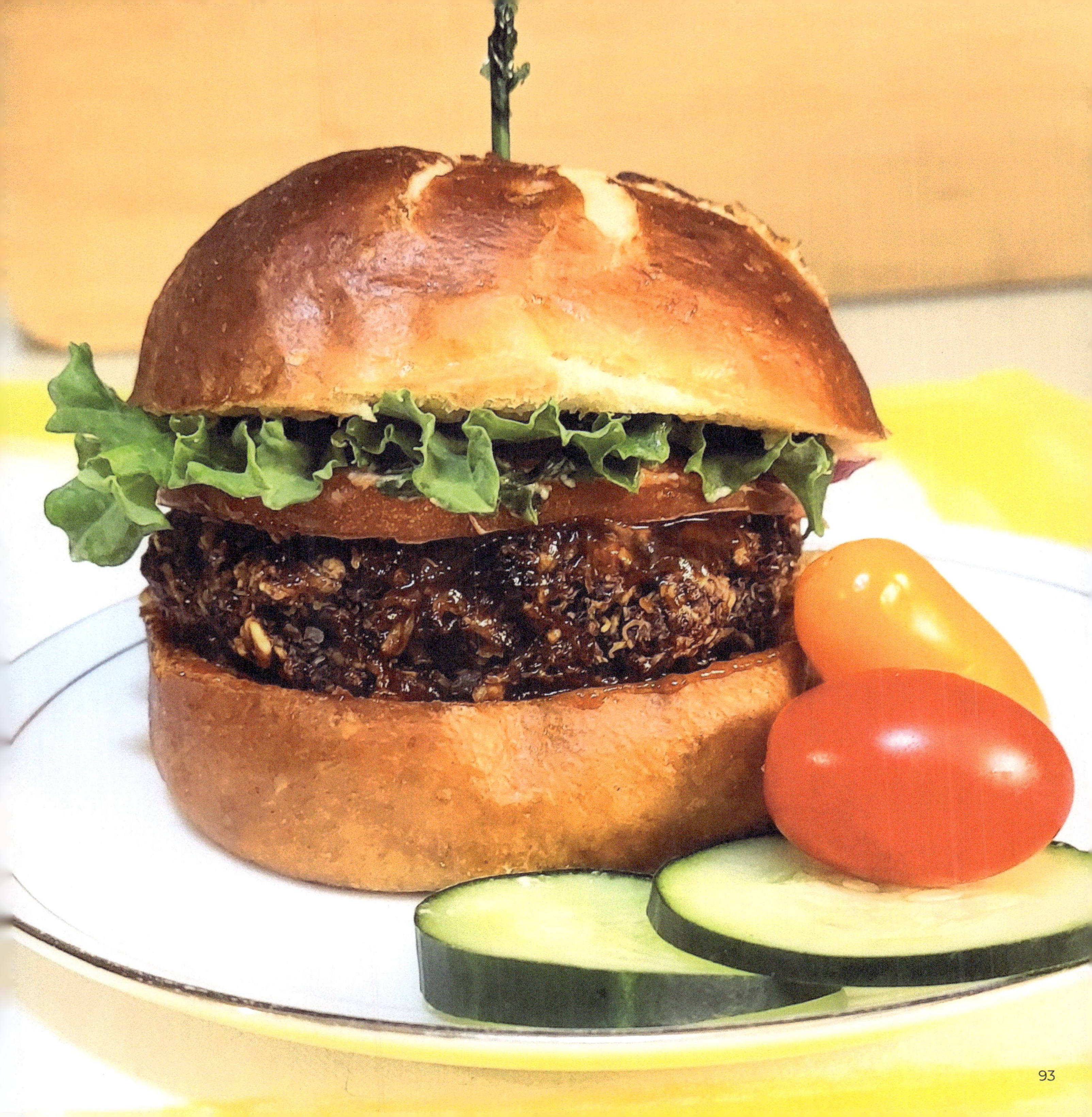

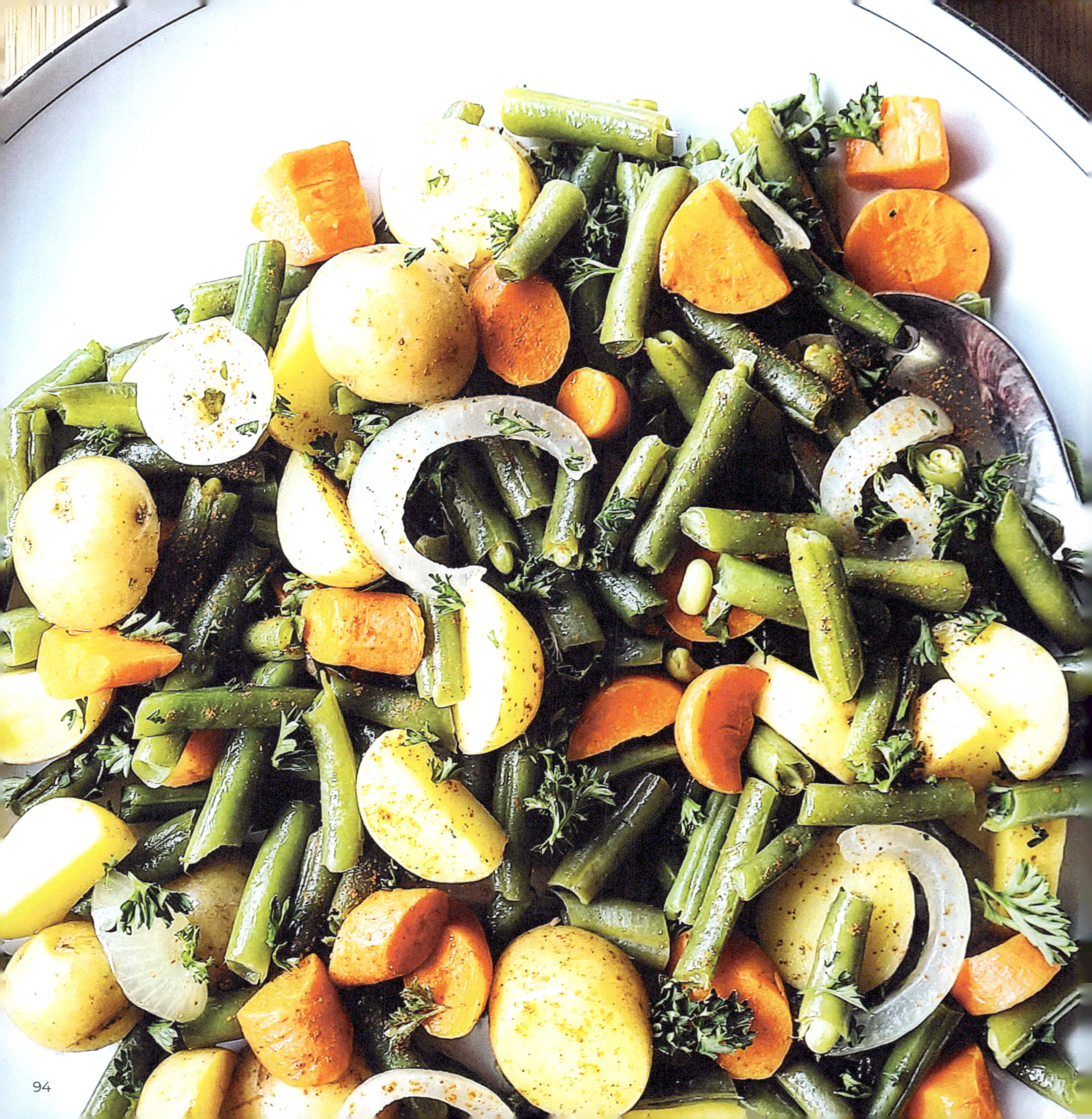

GREEN BEANS, POTATOES & CARROTS

When I was growing up, fresh string beans (green beans) always had a place at our Sunday dinner table. The sidekicks were potatoes and carrots. Because green beans were regulars on our plate, we grew up knowing how to "snap" string beans. But like most vegetables at that time, they were cooked for too long. In contrast, here I steam a pot of green beans with their "sidekicks" in a matter of just minutes.

String beans are a good source of copper, vitamin B1, chromium, magnesium, calcium, potassium, phosphorus, choline, vitamin A, and niacin.

INGREDIENTS:
2 pounds fresh green beans
3 carrots, scrubbed
3 large Yukon Gold or 6 petite gold potatoes, scrubbed and chopped
½ of a medium onion, sliced thinly
Drizzle of olive oil
½ cup parsley leaves, chopped
Sprinkling of cayenne pepper

PREPARATION:

1. Remove the ends from fresh green beans and snap beans into 2" pieces, then rinse well. Trim away ends of the carrots and chop carrots into chunks.
2. Add 3 cups of water into a saucepan, arrange vegetables - carrots first into the basket first, then the beans, potatoes and onions last, on the top. Cover steam basket and place over pot of boiling water. Steam vegetables until they are tender when pierced with a fork (approximately 15 minutes).
3. Remove the steam basket and drain the vegetables until no more water is dripping from them. Drizzle with oil and allow to drain a couple more minutes. Transfer vegetables to a bowl or large serving platter. Arrange vegetables and sprinkle with chopped parsley and pepper.

Makes 4 servings

TANGY BELL PEPPER - MUSHROOM WRAP

Slow simmered bell peppers, slivers of summer and zucchini squash, luscious mushrooms and fragrant onions come together quick and deliciously with new flavors and textures. Choose a wrap of your choice.

INGREDIENTS:

1-1/2 tablespoons coconut oil
1 medium onion (one cup)
3 bell peppers (green, red, yellow), julienne sliced
½ small summer squash, julienne sliced
½ small zucchini squash, julienne sliced
8 ounces button mushrooms, sliced
2 cloves of garlic, minced
1 teaspoon smoked paprika
1 teaspoon chili powder
2 teaspoons ground cumin
Sprinkle of black or white pepper
Handful of cilantro leaves
6 tortilla wraps or sliced bun

Optional Toppings: lime, salsa, beans, avocado, veggie cheese

PREPARATION:

1. Warm coconut oil in a medium- large skillet over low heat. Sauté onions, peppers and squash for 2 minutes. Stir in mushrooms and garlic, cover, and simmer over low heat for 3 additional minutes. Uncover and add spices, continue cooking uncovered until vegetables are fork tender but not mushy.

2. Scoop veggies onto a tortilla wrap or bun; finish with topping (s) and condiments of your choice

Makes 4 to 6 servings

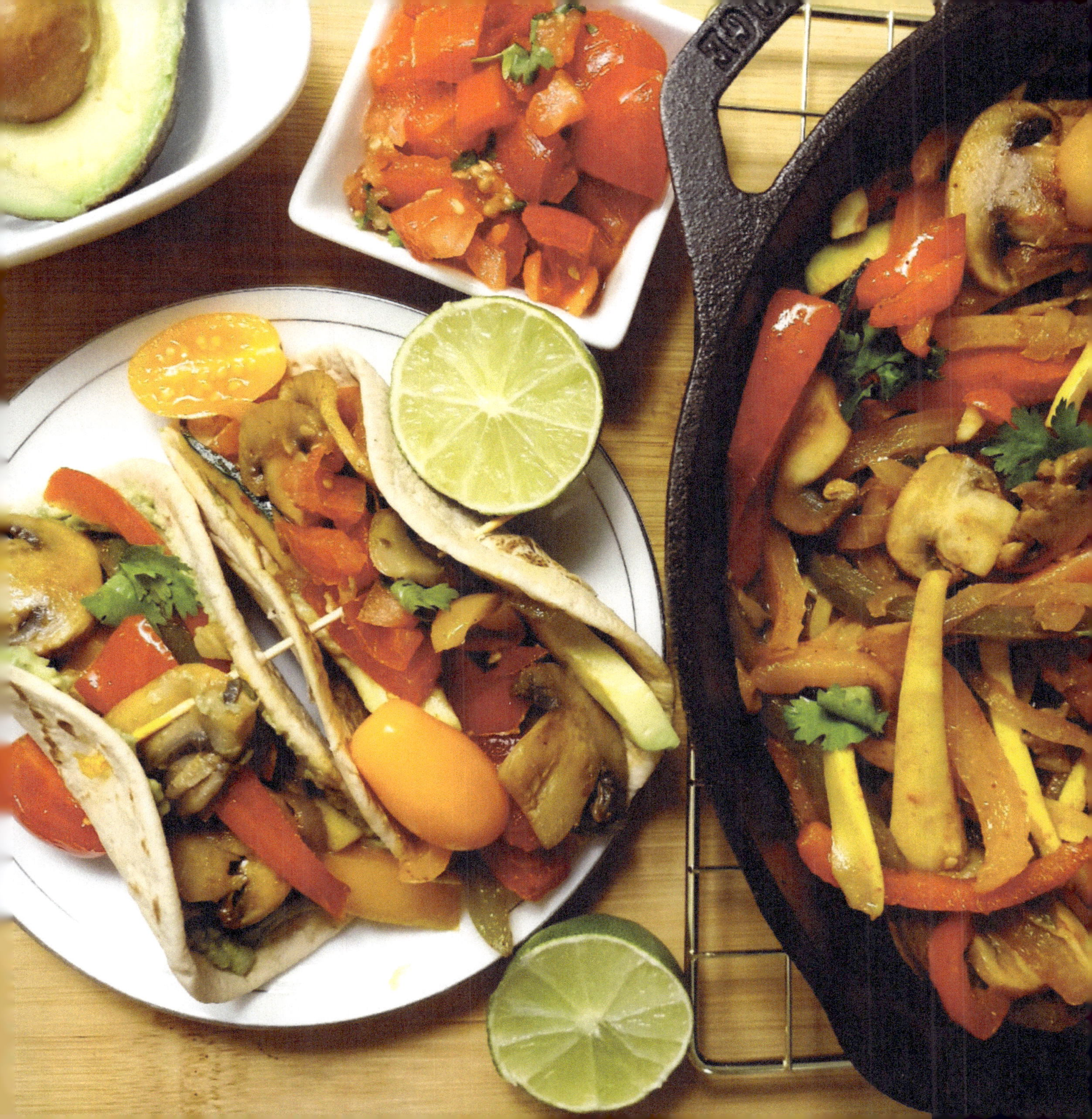

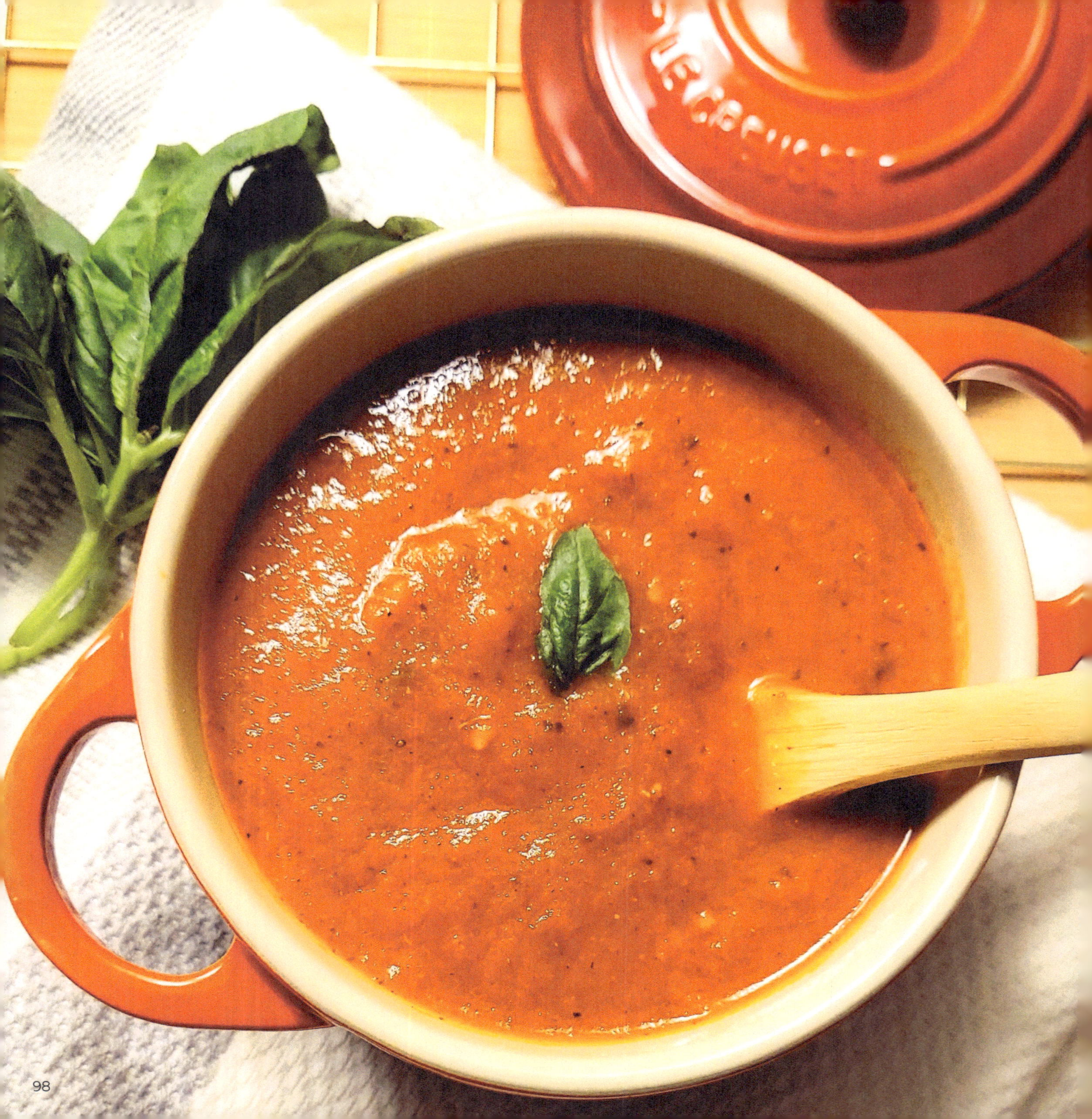

TOMATO SOUP

Tomatoes are the true taste of summer! Oh so wonderful in summer salads and numerous summer dishes. But don't forget Tomato Soup with the end -of-season ripe plum tomatoes. Plum tomatoes are more meaty and less water.

INGREDIENTS:

2 tablespoon olive oil
1-1/2 cups onion, chopped
3 cloves of garlic, diced
¼ teaspoon red pepper flakes
8 fully ripe plum tomatoes or
  1 - 28 ounce can peeled plum tomatoes, chopped
1 red bell pepper, chopped
1 teaspoon arrowroot + 1 teaspoon of soup
1 cup vegetable broth, store brought or homemade or (see recipe page 135)
½ teaspoon maple syrup (optional)
¼ teaspoon Celtic sea salt (optional)
1 cup fresh basil leaves or 1/3 cup of
  dried basil

PREPARATION:

1. Sauté onions in olive oil over low heat for 3 minutes. Add garlic cloves and red pepper flakes continue cooking for 2 additional minutes. Add tomatoes, red bell pepper. Mix arrow root and 1 teaspoon of soup in a small bowl until smooth, and stir into the soup. Cook for 25 minutes over a low heat, stirring frequently.

2. Stir in vegetable broth and cook for 5 minutes. Cut heat off and allow to cool. Taste, if the tomatoes are not sweet on their own, add a little sweetener and sea salt if you desire.

3. When soup is cool enough to pour, transfer to blender, add basil leaves. Blend on medium to high until smooth or add basil leaves and blend with handheld immersion blender.

Makes 24 ounces

STUFFED BELL PEPPERS

These bright peppers make a luscious and festive dish. This is a great side to prepare with leftover veggies, chopped greens and cooked quinoa or rice. Be creative with the veggies you have on hand.

INGREDIENTS:

4 bell peppers (any color)
½ tablespoon, coconut oil
1 small onion, diced
2 ribs celery, diced
2 cloves garlic, chopped
2 cups mushrooms, chopped
1 carrot, grated
1 cup cooked quinoa
2 teaspoons dried basil
2 teaspoons dried thyme
2 teaspoons smoked paprika
½ cup tomato sauce
Pepper and Celtic sea salt to taste
3 cups fresh spinach

PREPARATION: Preheat oven to 350°F.

1. Cut the peppers around the top and remove the seeds. Set aside.
2. Warm oil in a saucepan over medium-low heat. Add the onion and celery and sauté for 2 minutes. Add garlic, mushrooms and carrots and stir well. Reduce heat to low and cover for 2 minutes.
3. Stir in the quinoa, herbs, paprika, tomato sauce, celtic sea salt and pepper. Add the spinach, cover the pan and allow spinach to wilt. Fill the peppers with the quinoa mixture and arrange the stuffed peppers in an 8" square casserole dish. Add water to the dish and place in the oven. Bake for 25 minutes. Can be served with any leftover filling.

Makes 4 servings

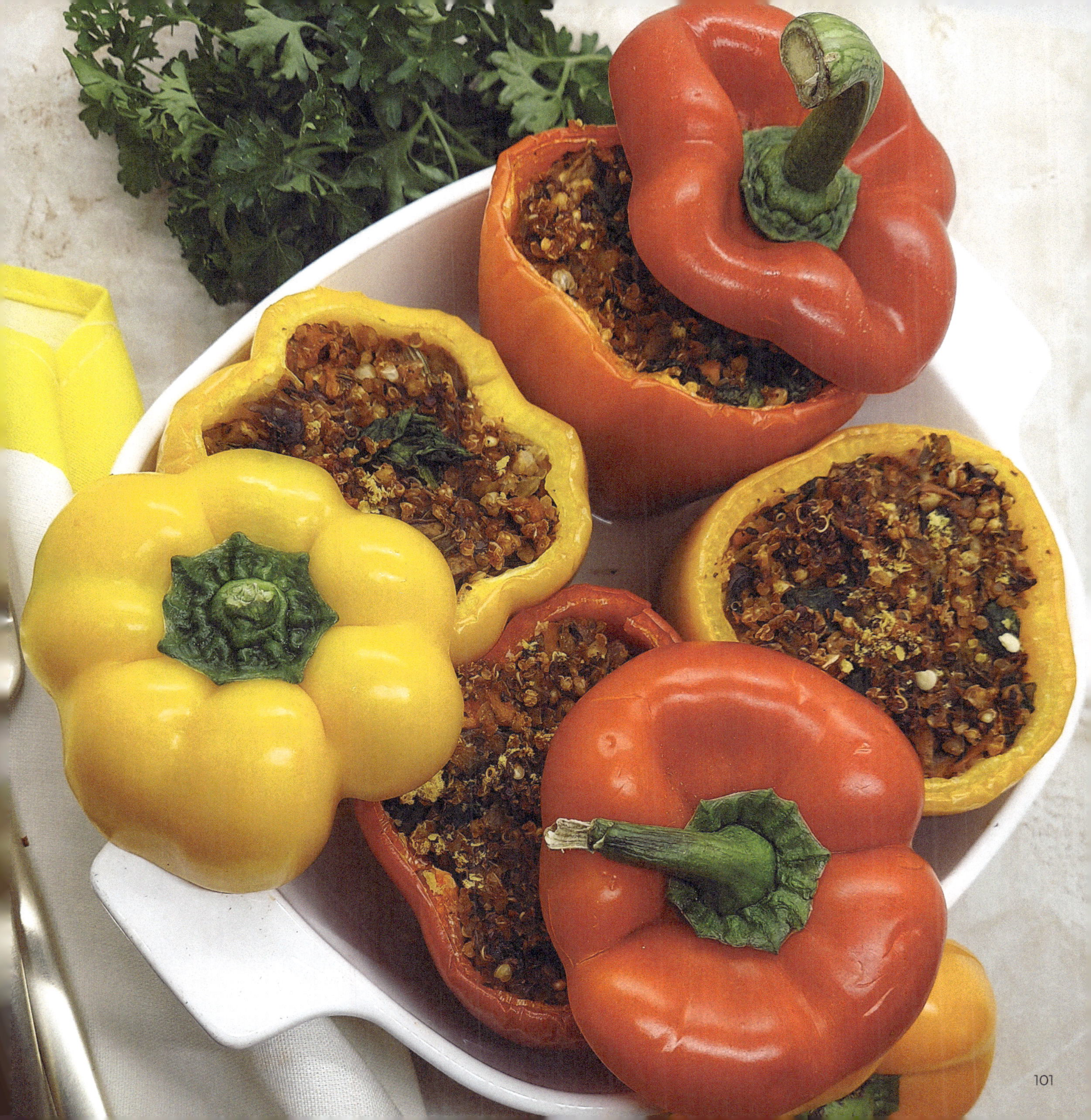

Fall Vegetables and Fruits

(partial listing)

Beets (Red)
Collard Greens
Kale
Mushrooms
Pumpkins
Red Potatoes
Sunchokes
Sweet Potatoes
Turnips
Winter Squash

Apples
Cranberries
Grapes
Pears
Persimmons

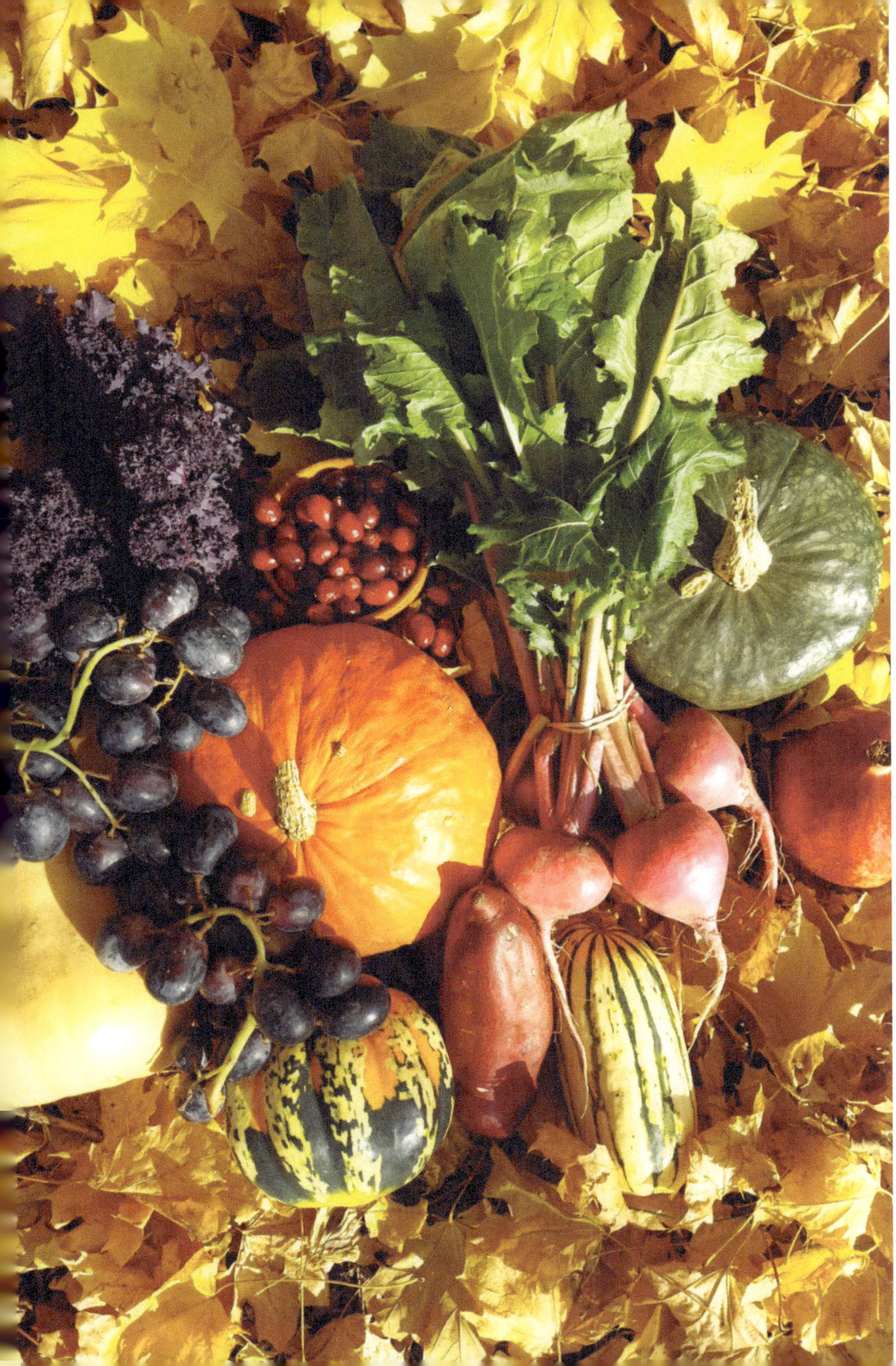

FALL

SEPTEMBER, OCTOBER + NOVEMBER

FALL RECIPES

The shift from summer to fall usually happens suddenly! First, there's a nip in the air; then comes windy days with cool nights; soon, leaves start changing color and falling from the trees. Our bodies also make seasonal shifts, and in many ways, so do our minds and emotions, also.

We can tell the season is changing when we notice the last of the summer tomatoes mixed in with the arrival of aromatic celery, colorful sweet potatoes and crisp apples. After those come the pumpkins, mushrooms, variety of winter squash and the rainbow of fall harvest colors.

At the farmer's market in the fall, we may also see a few cool season (spring and fall) crops returning - like spinach, beets, and swiss chard to name a few. Varieties of root vegetables such as beets and turnips—may arrive with their greens attached. Those intact greens are a double nutrient bonus! Beet and turnip greens are the most familiar. The greens or attached leaves are nutrient dense. I find myself going for the greens as much as for the more-familiar root vegetables.

Fall also brings great seasonal fruit, with multiple varieties of pears, apples and grapes, also persimmon a fruit worth exploring. Each season has its own individual brand and natural plan for our total health.

Let's welcome fall!

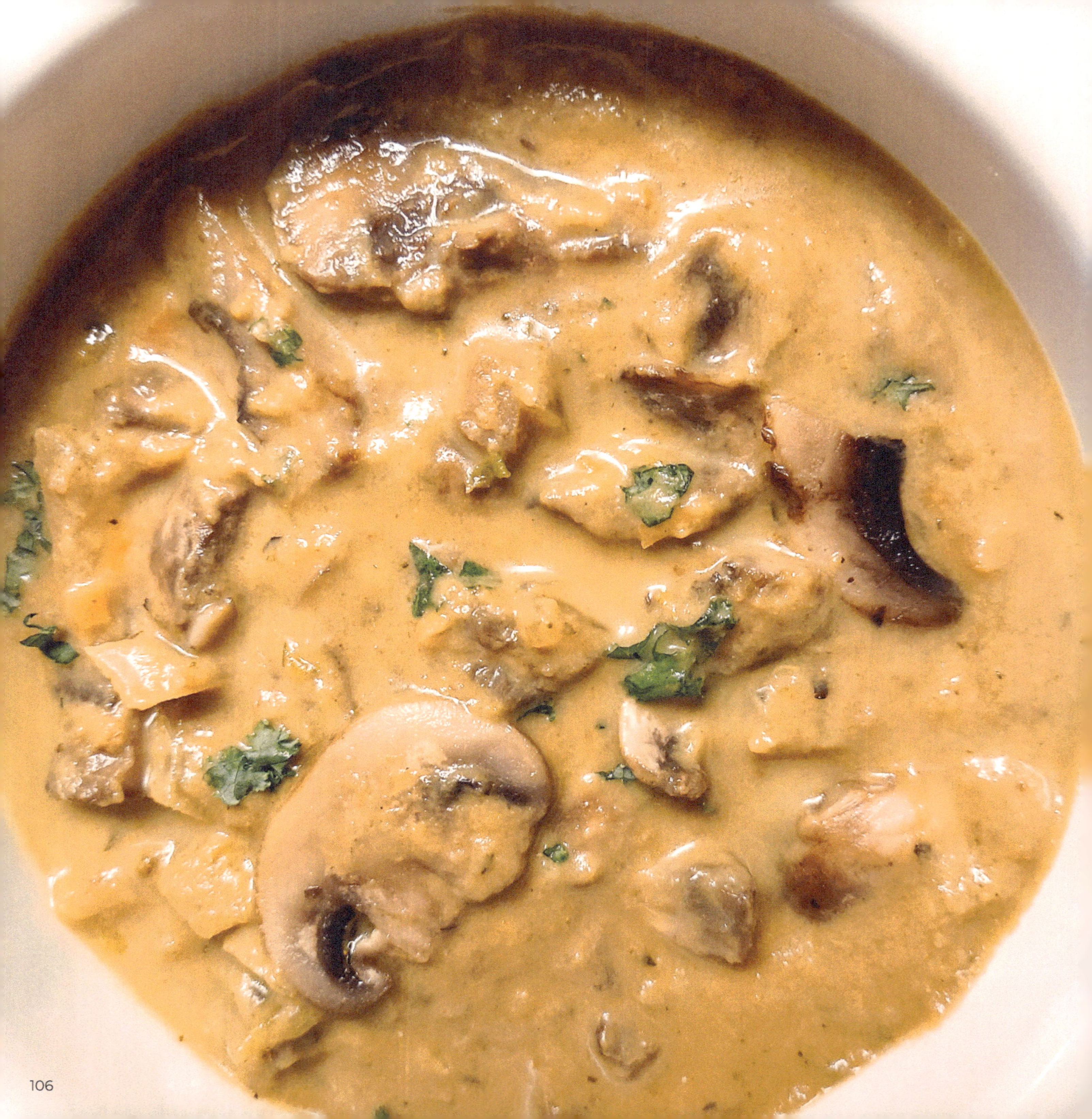

VEGAN MUSHROOM SOUP

This soup is worth its weight in nutrition and healing power. Mushrooms contain high levels of selenium, riboflavin (vitamin B2), pantothenic acid (vitamin B5), copper, potassium, and phosphorus. Cremini mushrooms are a good source of iron, and delightfully delicious!

INGREDIENTS:

2 tablespoon coconut oil, divided
1 onion, chopped
3 cloves garlic, minced
1 leek, white part only, thoroughly rinsed and then diced
1 large carrot, diced
2 ribs celery, diced
1-½ pounds cremini mushrooms, clean with a damp cloth and slice
1 tablespoon fresh lemon juice
½ teaspoon dried oregano
1 teaspoon dried thyme
¼ teaspoon each: ground coriander, cumin, and turmeric
½ teaspoon Celtic sea salt
½ teaspoon ground white pepper
1-½ cups vegetable broth + 2 teaspoons spelt flour or arrowroot (as a thickener)
1 cup unsweetened almond milk

PREPARATION:

1. Warm 1 tablespoon of coconut oil in a medium skillet over low heat. Add onions and sauté for 3 minutes. Stir in garlic, leek, carrot, and celery. Cook for 3 minutes, stirring occasionally. Cut off heat and cover.

2. Heat the remaining coconut oil in a large soup pot over very low heat. Add the mushrooms stir and cover pot, allow mushrooms to sweat in their own juice for 5 minutes. Add vegetable mixture to the mushrooms and stir in the lemon juice, herbs, spices, vegetable broth, salt, and pepper. Simmer 10 minutes

3. Spoon out ¼ cup of soup, add 2 teaspoons of spelt flour or arrowroot and blend until smooth. Stir into soup, add milk. Simmer for 20 minutes, remove the soup from the heat and allow to cool.

4. Pour half the soup into a blender, blend until smooth. Return the pureed soup to soup pot, give a good stir, warm and then cut off heat.

Makes 1 quart

PORTABELLA MUSHROOM STRIPS

Mushrooms really have more texture than taste. the meaty, firm texture of these mushrooms make a filling and delicious sandwich. Be creative, and add your favorite seasonings or a prepared sauce. The mushrooms will draw in the flavor.

INGREDIENTS:
1 teaspoon olive oil
1 medium onion, sliced thinly
1 clove garlic, diced
½ of a red bell pepper, sliced thinly
3 large portabella mushrooms, stems and gills removed, sliced thinly
5 button (or cremini) mushrooms, sliced
1 cup BBQ Sauce (see page 200)
4 rolls or buns, sliced in half

PREPARATION:

1. Warm the olive oil in a large skillet over medium heat. Add the onion, garlic, bell pepper, and mushrooms. Cover and reduce heat to low. Allow to sweat for 5-7 minutes.

2. Uncover and simmer until all liquid has cooked into the mushrooms. Stir in the BBQ sauce and stir well to combine. Simmer over very low heat until fragrant and brown.

3. Place a generous scoop of mushrooms and peppers onto the buns, add more sauce, cover and enjoy.

Makes 4 servings

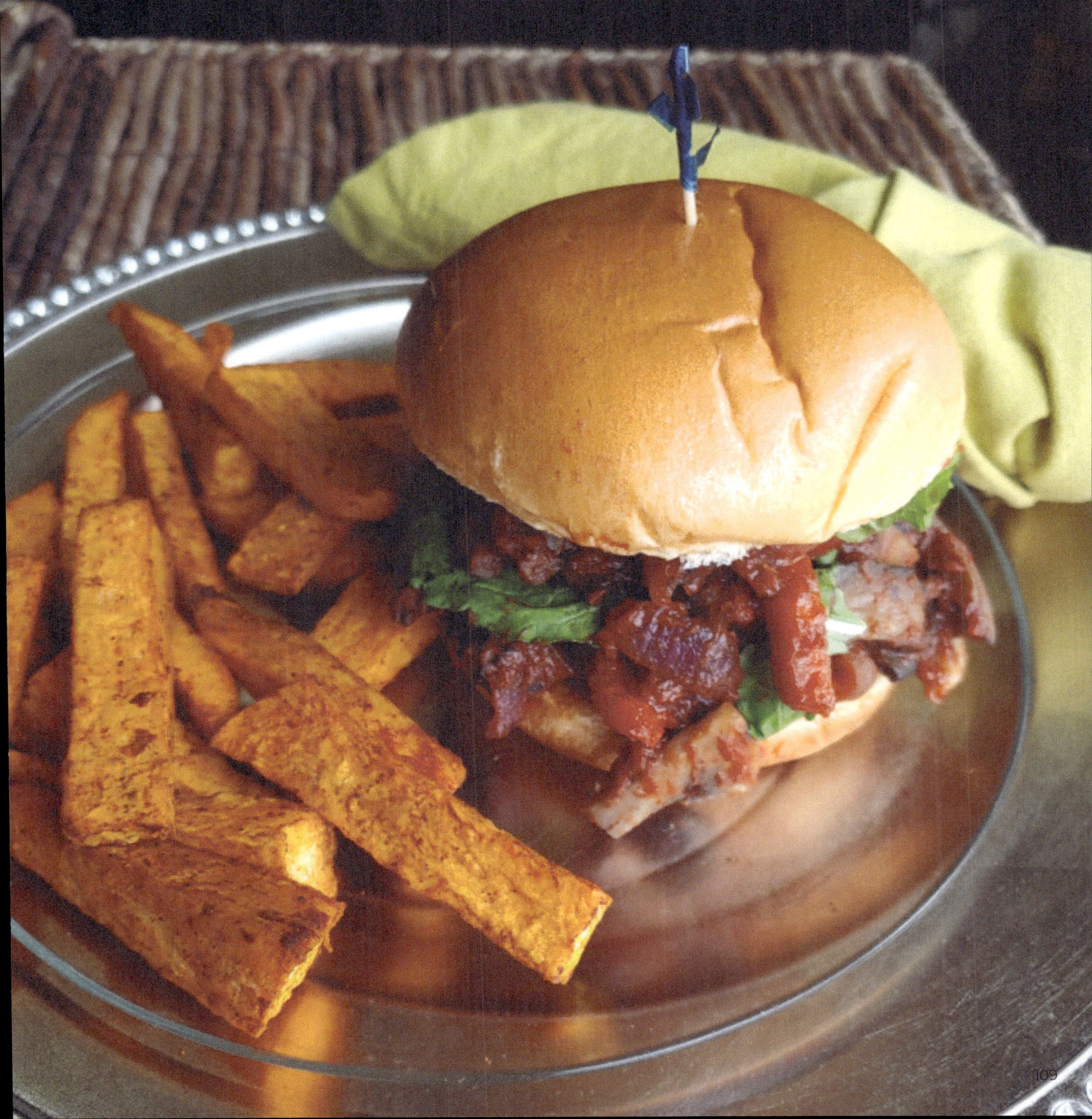

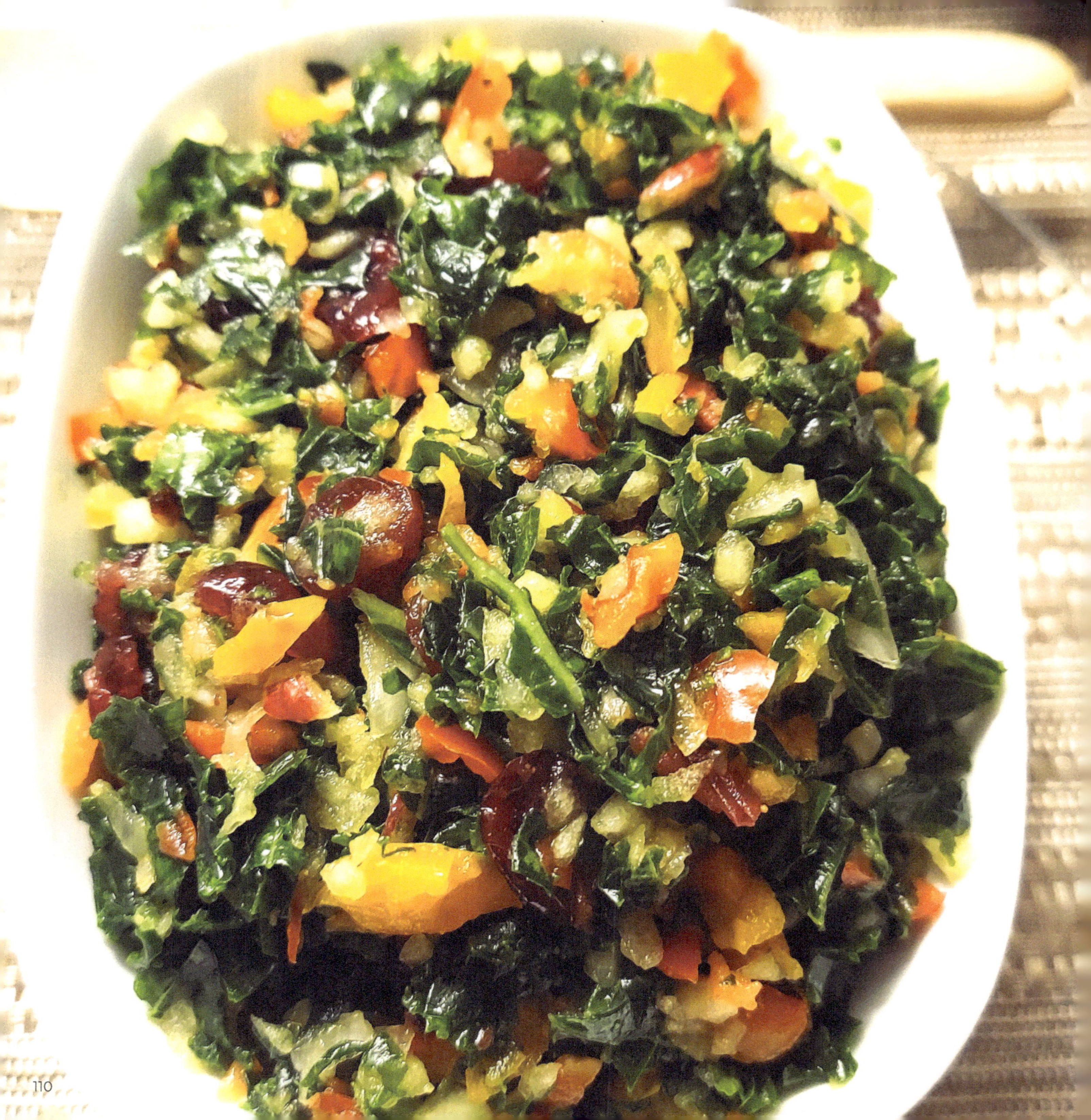

KALE SALAD SUPREME

This super salad is very versatile when it comes to using seasonal ingredients. In the fall, apples and in the winter, pomegranates are a tasty, healthy option. Dark green leafy vegetables are said to be the healthiest plants on the planet. (Note: Taking medication can limit your intake of green vegetables. Consult your healthcare provider/practitioner.)

INGREDIENTS:

1 bunch curly kale leaves, stems removed, leaves wash and dried
1 tablespoon lemon juice
1 tablespoon olive oil
½ of a medium onion, diced (about ½ cup)
½ of a red bell pepper, diced
1 peeled apple, grated
Dash of ground ginger
½ cup dried unsweetened cranberries
Pinch of Celtic sea salt

PREPARATION:

1. Chop the kale into small pieces. Add the lemon juice and olive oil and massage the kale with your fingers for about 3 minutes until the leaves are soft and pliable.

2. Place the massaged kale in a salad bowl. Fluff the kale with a fork. Stir in the onion, red pepper, grated apple, ginger, and cranberries. Toss well to blend. Taste and add Celtic sea salt as needed.

3. Cover and refrigerate.

Makes 4 servings

SWEET POTATO CURRY

For this curry recipe, we are simmering sweet potatoes and sweet bell peppers in a handcrafted curry sauce. The spices and potatoes are warming and appetizing! The recipe can be doubled or served as a side.

INGREDIENTS:

1 tablespoon coconut oil
1 small onion, chopped (½cup)
2 teaspoons fresh ginger, minced
(or 1 teaspoon ground)
3 cloves garlic, minced
One 28-ounce can of whole
plum tomatoes, chopped
1 teaspoon fresh lime juice
½ teaspoon dried thyme
1 teaspoon ground cumin
1 teaspoon ground coriander
1 teaspoon curry powder
½ teaspoon ground turmeric
¼ teaspoon ground cloves
Dash of cayenne pepper
15 ounces whole coconut milk
½ teaspoon Celtic sea salt
2 sweet potatoes, peeled and chopped
½ of a bell pepper, green or red,
chopped

PREPARATION:

1. In a large skillet over low heat, warm coconut oil. Add the onions, ginger and garlic and cook for 2 minutes.
2. Stir in the tomatoes, thyme, spices and lime juice. Add the coconut milk and add salt as you desire.
3. Add the sweet potatoes and peppers and reduce the heat to low. Cook, stirring occasionally, for 30 minutes or until the potatoes are tender when pierced with a fork.

Makes 4 servings

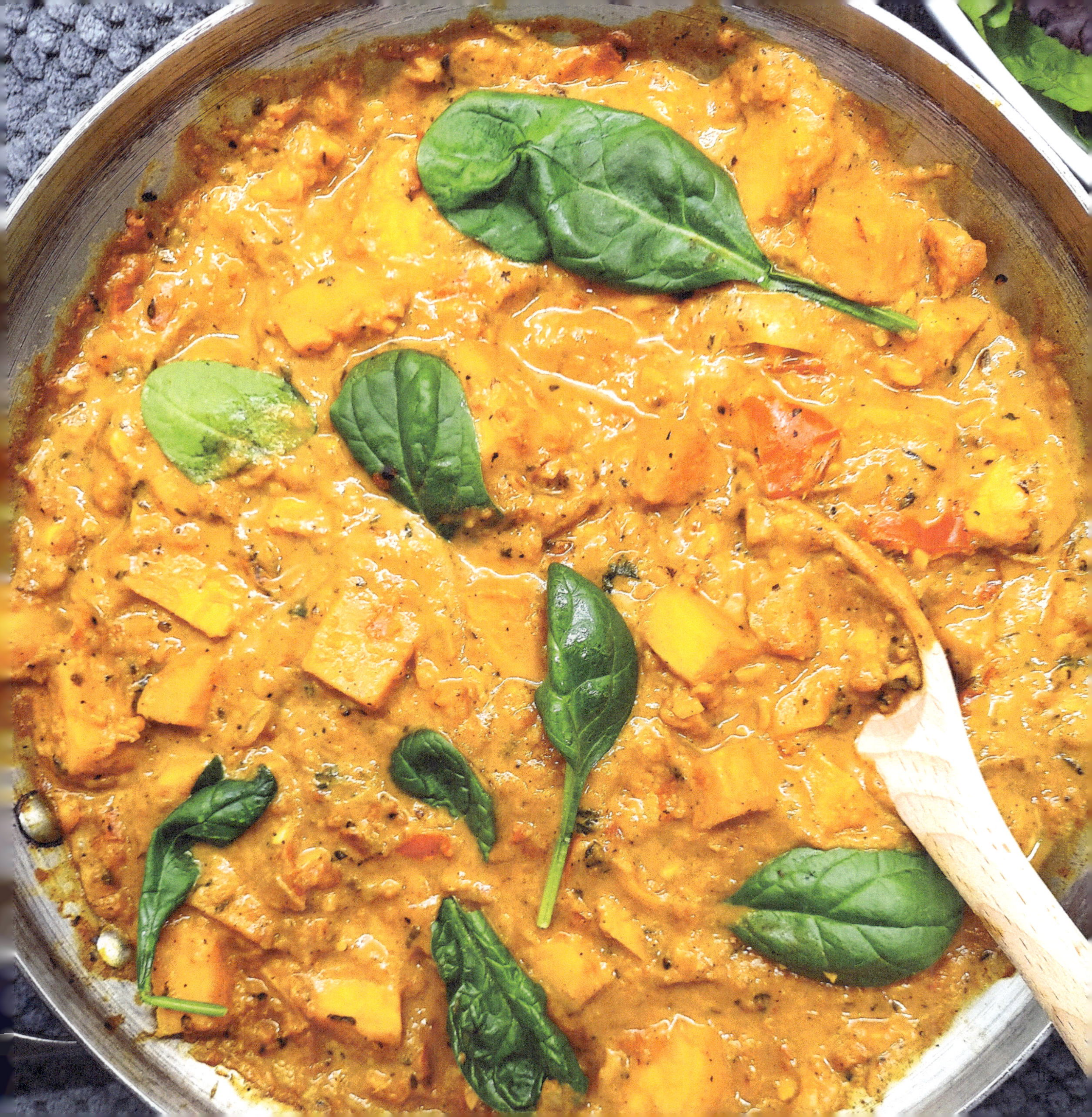

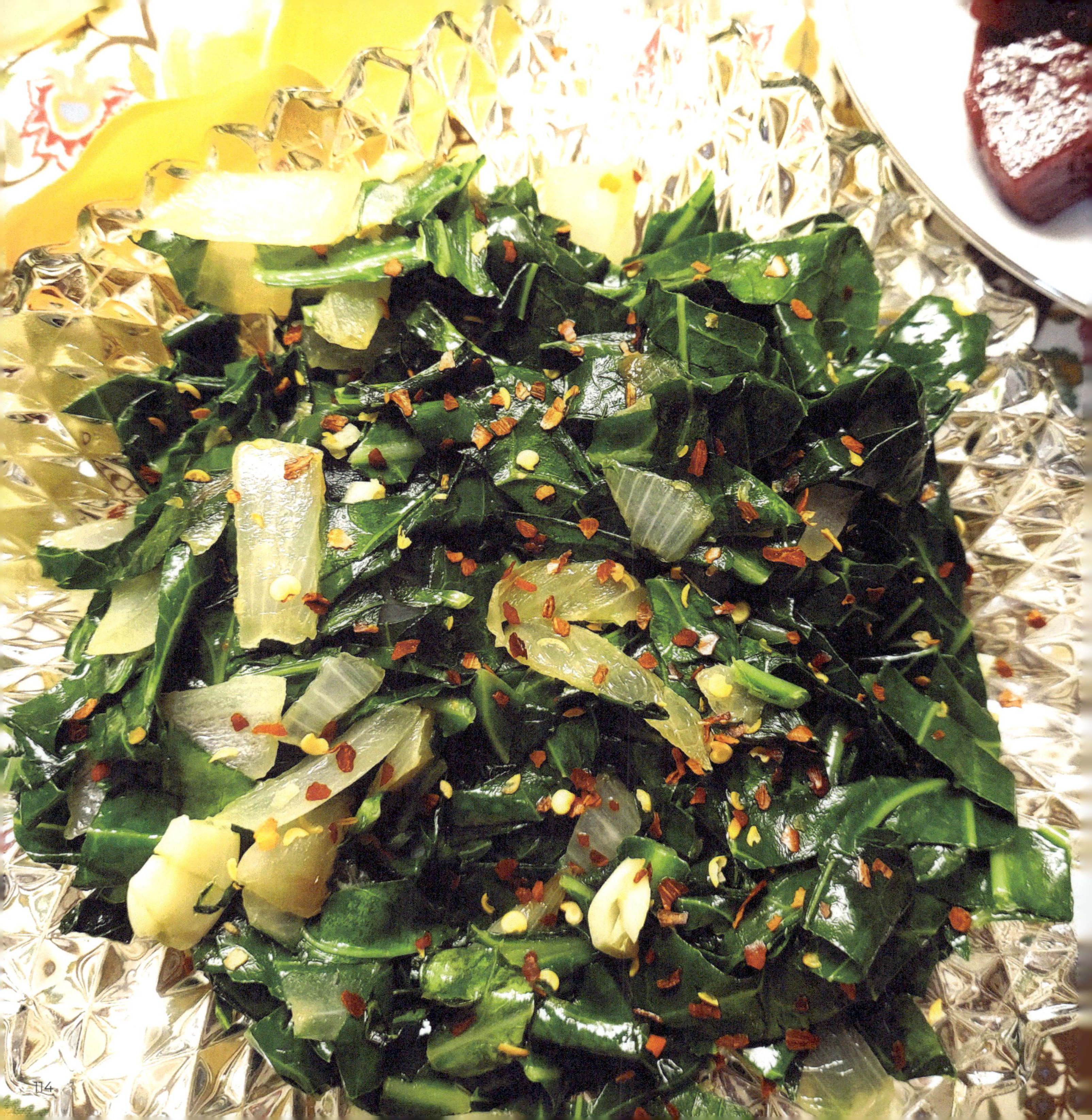

SAUTEED COLLARD GREENS

Growing up, I always heard that "greens" (collards, mustard greens, turnip greens) tasted best after the frost hit them. I also remember that they were cooked all day long. In this recipe, however, the collards take a minimum amount of time to cook in a heavy-bottomed skillet or wok.

INGREDIENTS:

2 bunches collard greens, washed, stems removed
1 tablespoon coconut oil
1 small onion, chopped
3 cloves garlic, minced
1 teaspoon smoked paprika
1 teaspoon ground ginger
½ teaspoon red pepper flakes
Celtic sea salt and black pepper to taste

PREPARATION:

1. Roll the collard leaves into cylinders and cut into ribbons. (This is called a chiffonade cut)
2. Warm the coconut oil in a large, heavy-bottomed skillet or wok over low heat. Add the onion and sauté for 2 minutes, then add the garlic and continue cooking until the onion is soft.
3. Add the collards and sprinkle in the ginger, red pepper flakes and 1 cup of water. Cover and simmer for 20 minutes or until tender. If the pan gets dry before the collards are done, add water and keep cooking. Salt and black pepper to taste.

Makes 4 servings

FRESH CRANBERRY SAUCE

This is an easy cranberry sauce made from real, whole cranberries. Purchase whole cranberries in autumn, when they are in season and readily available, and store them in the freezer to use in smoothies, sauces, or baked goods throughout the year.

INGREDIENTS:

12 ounces fresh cranberries
Juice and zest of 1 orange
½ cup water
¼ cup maple syrup
1 teaspoon ground cinnamon

PREPARATION:

1. Place all ingredients in a medium-size saucepan and bring to a boil. Reduce the heat to low and allow the cranberries to simmer for 20 minutes or until the berries pop open, soften, and start to thicken.
2. Let cool and thicken at room temperature for 30 minutes before serving or refrigerate for later use.

Makes 3 cups

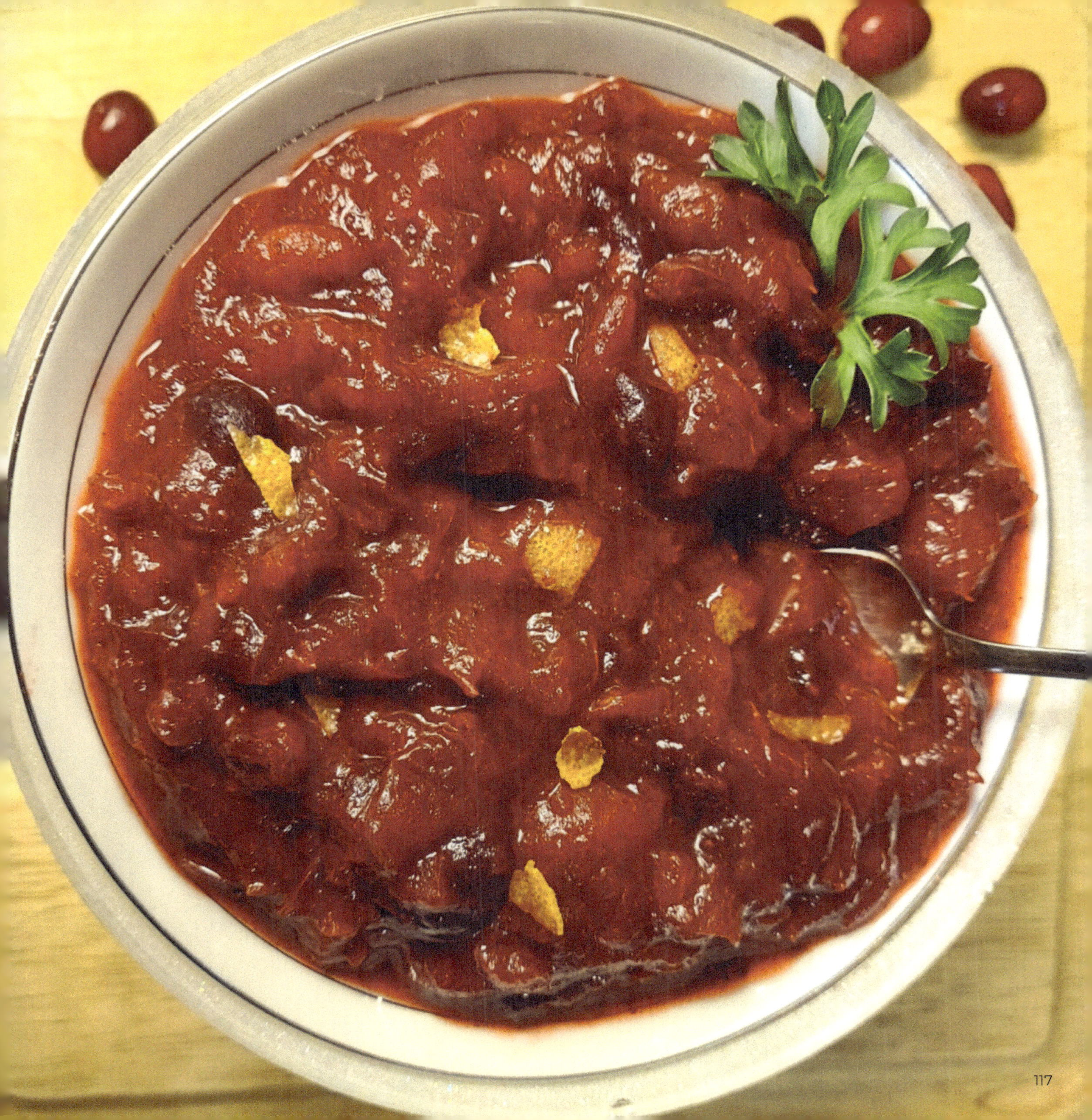

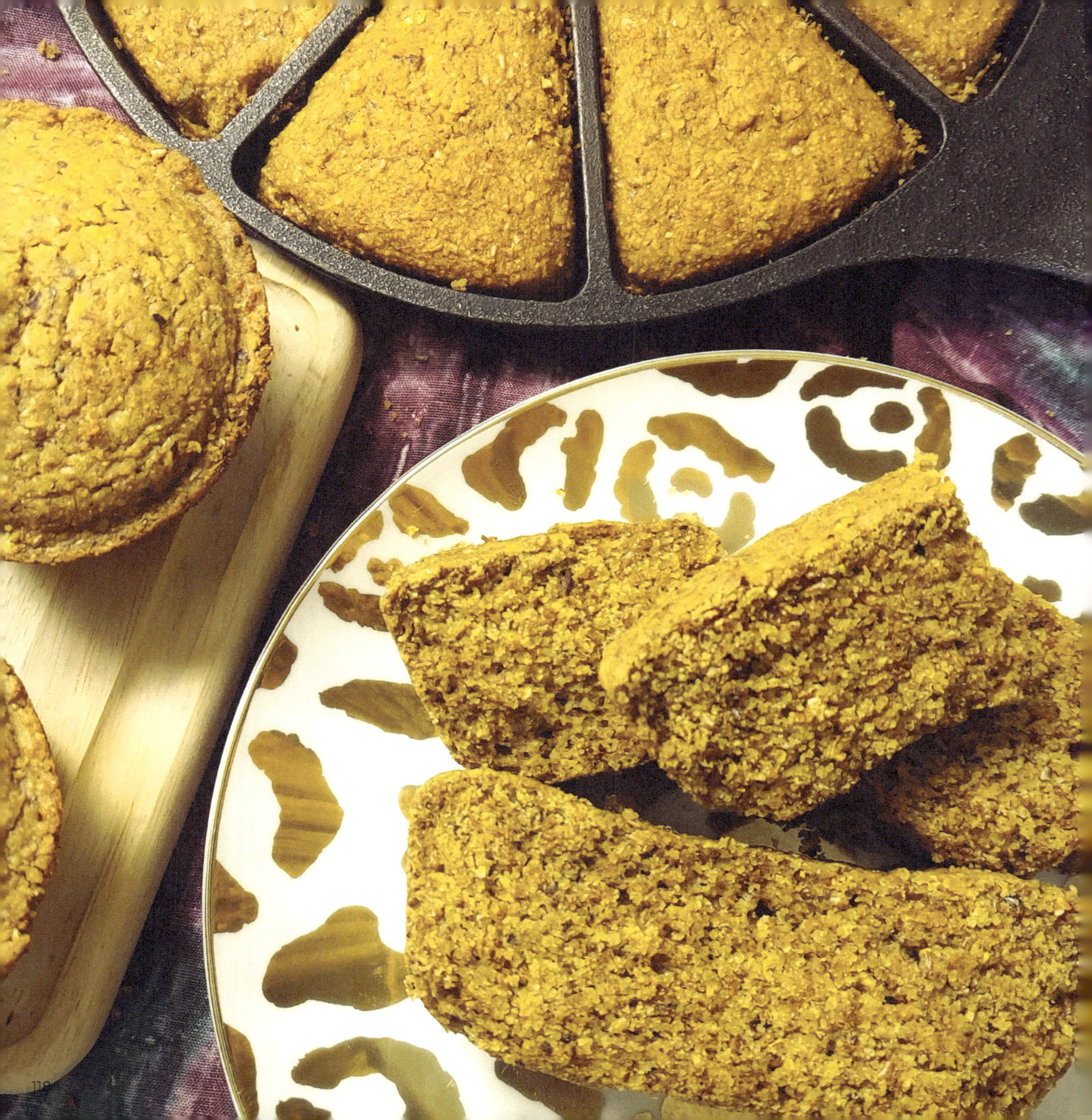

BEV'S VEGAN CORNBREAD

The secret to this awesome cornbread is the organic cornmeal. (Organic is non-GMO by definition.) The quality of the cornmeal makes all the difference in this cornbread and the cornbread dressing.

INGREDIENTS:
1 tablespoon ground flaxseeds
1 cup organic cornmeal
1 cup spelt flour
1 tablespoon aluminum-free baking powder
½ teaspoon baking soda
½ teaspoon Celtic sea salt
1 cup non-dairy milk
¼ cup maple syrup
1/3 cup olive oil

PREPARATION: Preheat oven to 400°F. Oil a cast-iron skillet or baking pan.

1. In a small bowl, mix the ground flaxseeds with 3 tablespoons of water. Let stand for 3 minutes to thicken.

2. In a medium-size mixing bowl, blend the dry ingredients. In another bowl, whisk together the milk, maple syrup, and oil. Add the flaxseed mixture.

3. Place the oiled skillet or pan in the oven for 3 minutes. Pour the wet ingredients into the dry ingredients and mix together until just combined. Remove the hot skillet/pan from the oven and pour in the batter immediately. Return the pan to the oven and bake for 30 minutes or until an inserted toothpick comes out clean and dry.

Makes 6 to 8 servings

BEV'S VEGAN CORNBREAD DRESSING

This is a classic side dish made from vegan cornbread. It still receives raves! (Yes, I continue to refer to this dish as "dressing" even though it is not used to dress or stuff anything.)

INGREDIENTS:

1 onion, diced
1 tablespoon olive oil
4 ounces cremini or button mushrooms, clean with a damp cloth and chopped
1 rib celery, diced
½ of a green bell pepper, diced
2 cups vegetable broth or water
2 tablespoons dried sage, divided
½ teaspoon dried rosemary
½ teaspoon dried thyme
½ teaspoon dried oregano
1 pan cornbread (see page 119)
1/8 teaspoon ground coriander
1/8 teaspoon ground cumin
1/8 teaspoon ground turmeric
Celtic sea salt and pepper to taste

PREPARATION: Preheat oven to 375°F. Oil a baking casserole dish/pan.

1. In a medium saucepan over low heat, add the oil, onion, mushrooms, celery, and green pepper. Pour in the stock or water.
2. Simmer for 10 minutes. Stir in 1 tablespoon of sage along with the rosemary, thyme, and oregano. Continue simmering on very low heat for another 10 minutes.
3. Crumble the cornbread into a large mixing bowl. Fluff with your hands. Add the cooked vegetables, the remaining tablespoon of sage, the remaining spices, the Celtic sea salt and pepper. Mix well. Add more stock (as needed) to moisten the mixture.
4. Pour the dressing into the oiled baking casserole dish/pan and bake for 30 minutes or until the dressing is firm and an inserted tooth pick comes out clean.

Makes 6 to 8 servings

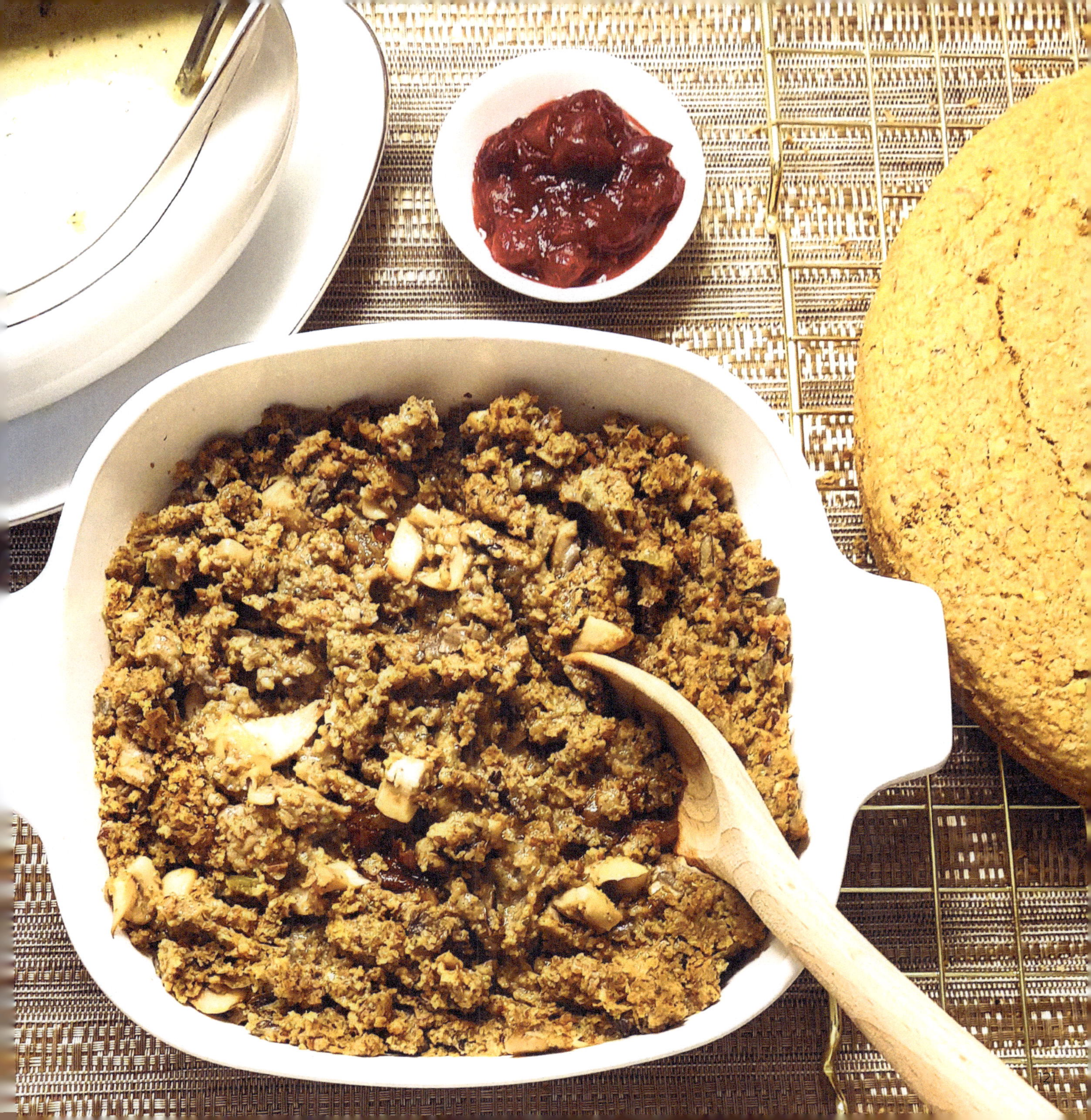

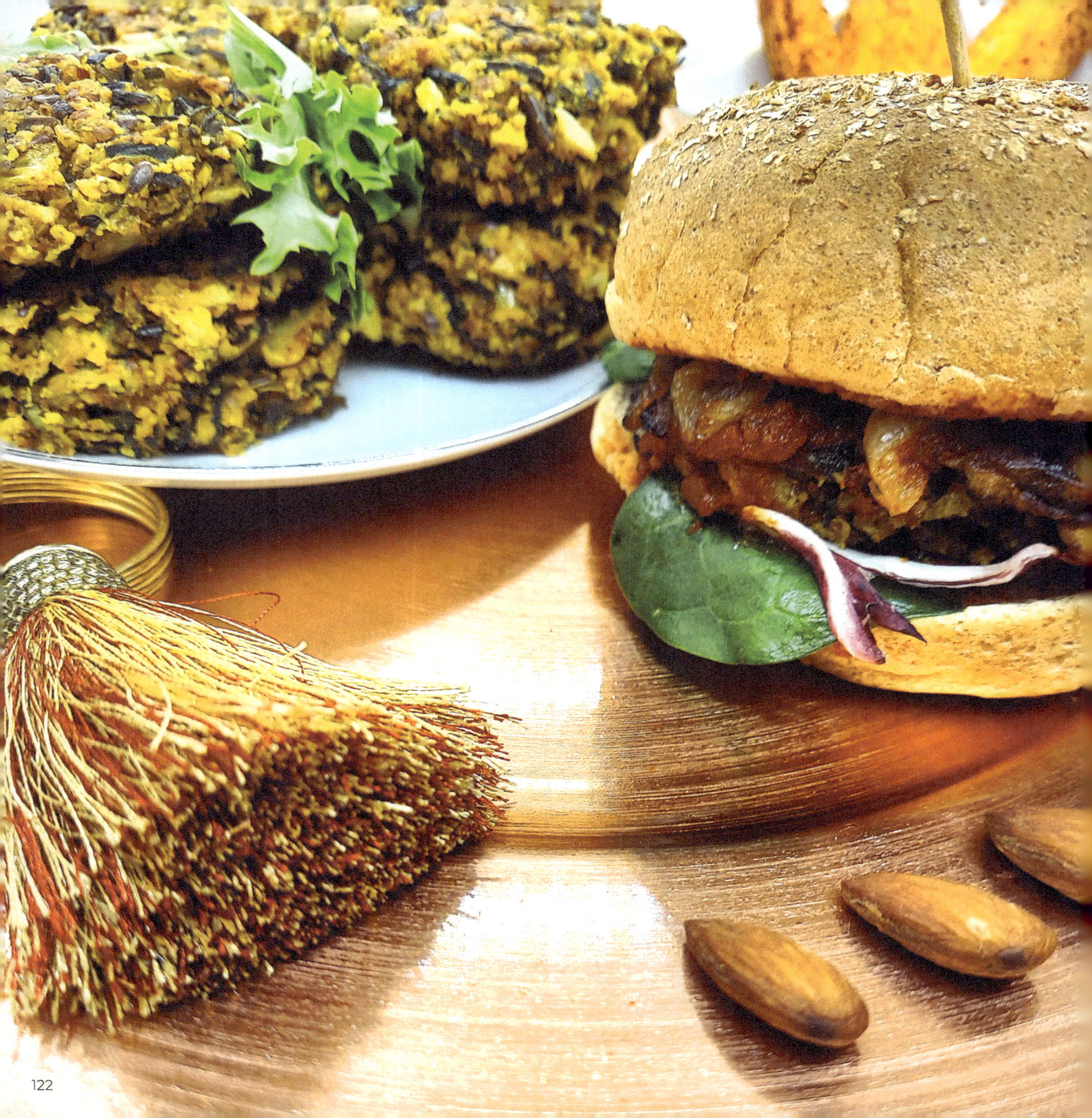

WILD RICE AND ALMOND SLIDERS

These wonderful sliders were created when wild rice was the only grain I was eating. My first thought was, "What to do with wild rice?" This burger creation was my answer. It was the perfect way to enjoy the chewy, nutty wild rice and to benefit from the nutrition packed into this amazing seed of an aquatic grass. I hope you enjoy it, too!

INGREDIENTS:

1 tablespoon ground flaxseeds
1 cup wild rice
1 cup raw almonds
3 cloves garlic, minced
1 onion, minced
1 teaspoon smoked paprika
1 teaspoon ground turmeric
1 teaspoon ground cumin
1 teaspoon dried thyme
Celtic sea salt to taste
Dash of cayenne pepper
4 slider buns

PREPARATION: Preheat oven to 350°F.

1. Place the ground flaxseeds in a small bowl and add 3 tablespoons of water. Stir and let stand to thicken.
2. Rinse wild rice thoroughly. Place in a large pot with 3½ cups of water. Bring to a boil over medium heat. Once boiling, lower heat, cover and simmer until the kernels split open (30 minutes). Drain in a colander, use back of spoon to press out excess water.
3. While rice is cooking, place almonds in a small, dry skillet and toast, stir often, over medium heat for 4-5 minutes. Watch almonds during this time! Toast until slightly golden and very fragrant. Once cool grind them into a coarse flour.
4. Transfer the cooked rice to a large bowl. While still warm, fold in the garlic and onion. Add the flaxseed mixture, spices, thyme, salt, and pepper and combine well. Mix in the ground almonds.
5. Form the rice-almond mixture into 4 patties and place them on a baking sheet lined with parchment paper. Bake for 15 minutes on each side. Serve on buns with condiments of your choice.

Makes 4 sliders

BUTTERNUT, CARROT AND APPLE BISQUE

I use the term "bisque" to indicate that this soup is thicker than typical soup. The rich flavor of butternut squash combined with carrots and apples makes it a velvety, warm treat. Carrots and butternut squash contain plentiful amounts of beta-carotene and antioxidants! I have also thin it out and served it as a gravy.

INGREDIENTS:

1 tablespoon coconut oil
1 sweet yellow onion, chopped
2 carrots, chopped
1 apple, chopped
4 cups vegetable broth
1 medium butternut squash, peel, seeds removed, cut into chunks
¼ teaspoon ground nutmeg
¼ teaspoon ground ginger
1 teaspoon curry powder
½ teaspoon ground cinnamon
¼ teaspoon Celtic sea salt
1/8 teaspoon black pepper
½ cup whole coconut milk
Optional: 1 teaspoon of sweetener of your choice

PREPARATION:

1. Warm the coconut oil in a large soup pot over low heat. Add the onion and sauté for 2 minutes. Stir in the carrots and apple and sauté the mixture for 3 minutes.
2. Add the broth, squash, spices, salt, and pepper and cover the pot. Continue cooking over medium-low heat for 30 minutes or until the vegetables are soft. Remove from the heat and let cool.
3. Carefully pour the cooled soup into a blender and blend (or blend with an immersion blender) until smooth. Return the soup to the pot. Stir in the coconut milk and sweetener (if desired) and simmer over medium heat for 10 minutes.

Makes 4 cups

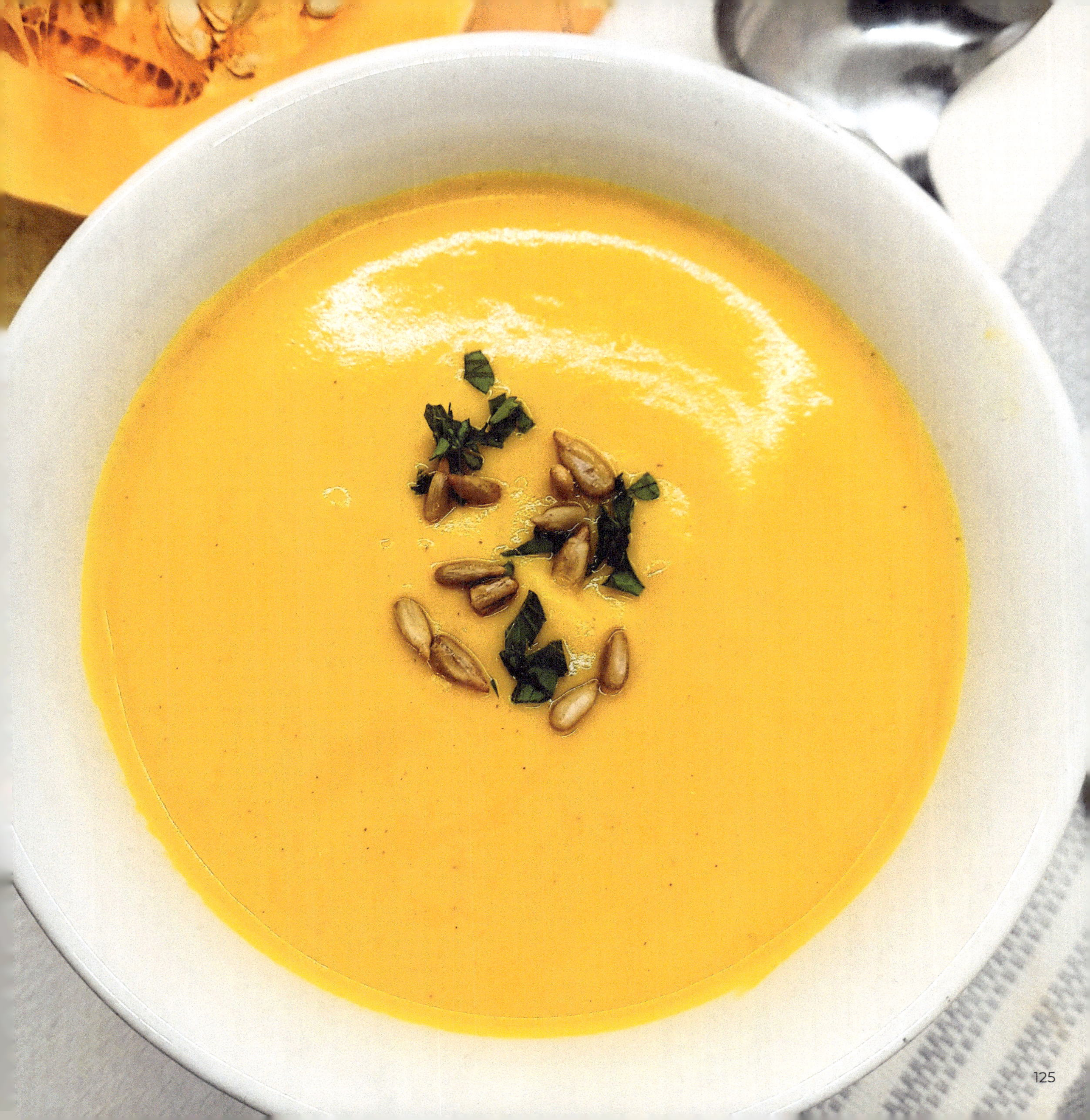

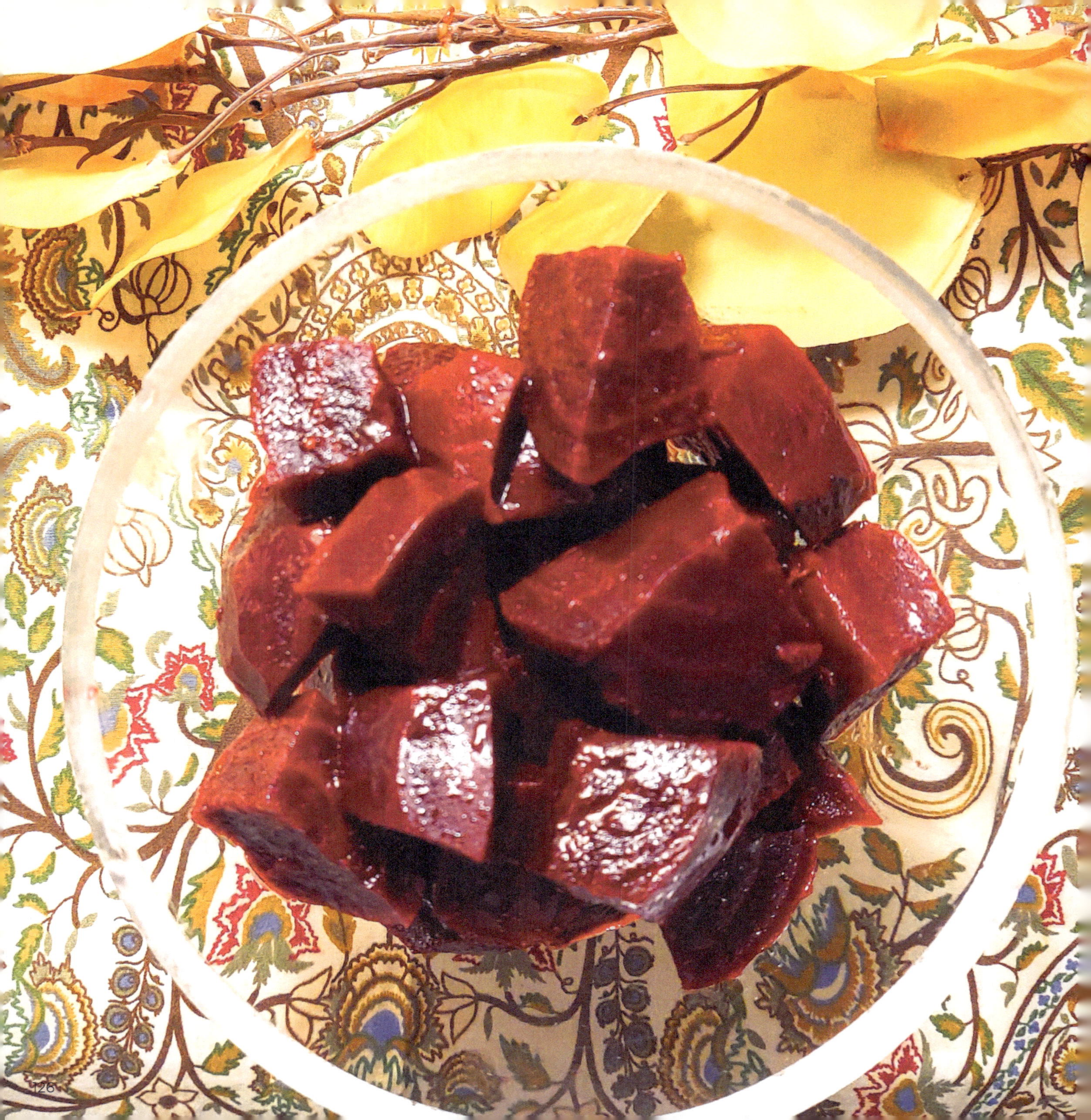

MARINATED RED BEETS

This marinade brings out the earthy essence of red beets. Beets are a good source of potassium and vitamin C. Serve as an appetizer, a side, or on a salad. The edible beet greens are high in beta-carotene. These greens can also substitute for Swiss chard or spinach.

INGREDIENTS:

1 bunch red beets, organic when possible
Juice of 1 orange
2 tablespoons walnut oil or olive oil
2 tablespoon balsamic vinegar

PREPARATION:

1. Wash beets, trim the tops, leave a 3" stem on bottom. Add water to a medium-size pot. Place beets in a steam basket, over the pot and cover. Steam for 20 minutes or until beets are fork-tender. Once cool, the beet skins will peel off easily. Cut beets into chunks.

2. Whisk together orange juice, the oil and vinegar. Add the beets to the marinade, stir well to coat, and cover. Refrigerate for at least 15 minutes before serving. Beets can be stored in the refrigerator for up to a week.

Makes 2 to 3 servings

VEGETARIAN CHILI

This hearty vegetarian chili is best made with dried beans rather than canned beans — the bean gravy that develops from cooking the dried beans is what truly sets this dish apart.

INGREDIENTS:

1 pound dried kidney beans, soaked overnight
1 tablespoon olive oil
1 onion, diced
2 ribs celery, diced
3 cloves garlic, minced
1 carrot, chopped
3½ cups vegetable broth
2 bay leaves
One 28-ounce can of diced plum tomatoes
1 teaspoon dried oregano
1 teaspoon dried basil
2 teaspoons ground cumin
2 teaspoons smoked paprika
2 tablespoons chili powder
Celtic sea salt to taste
Dash of cayenne pepper
½ of a green bell pepper, chopped
½ of a red bell pepper, chopped

PREPARATION: Cover the dry beans in water and soak overnight. The next day, drain and rinse them well.

1. In a large soup pot over medium-low heat, warm the oil. Add onions, celery, garlic, and carrot and sauté in olive oil for 3 minutes, stirring occasionally. Add the broth, bay leaves and beans, and bring to a rapid boil over medium heat. Reduce heat to low and simmer for 20 minutes.

2. Add the tomatoes, herbs, spices, salt, and pepper then stir in the bell peppers and continue on simmer for 15 minutes.

3. By now, the chili will have thickened and the bell peppers should be tender to the touch of a fork. Add water if the chili is getting thicker than you want. Remove the bay leaves before serving.

Makes 4 servings

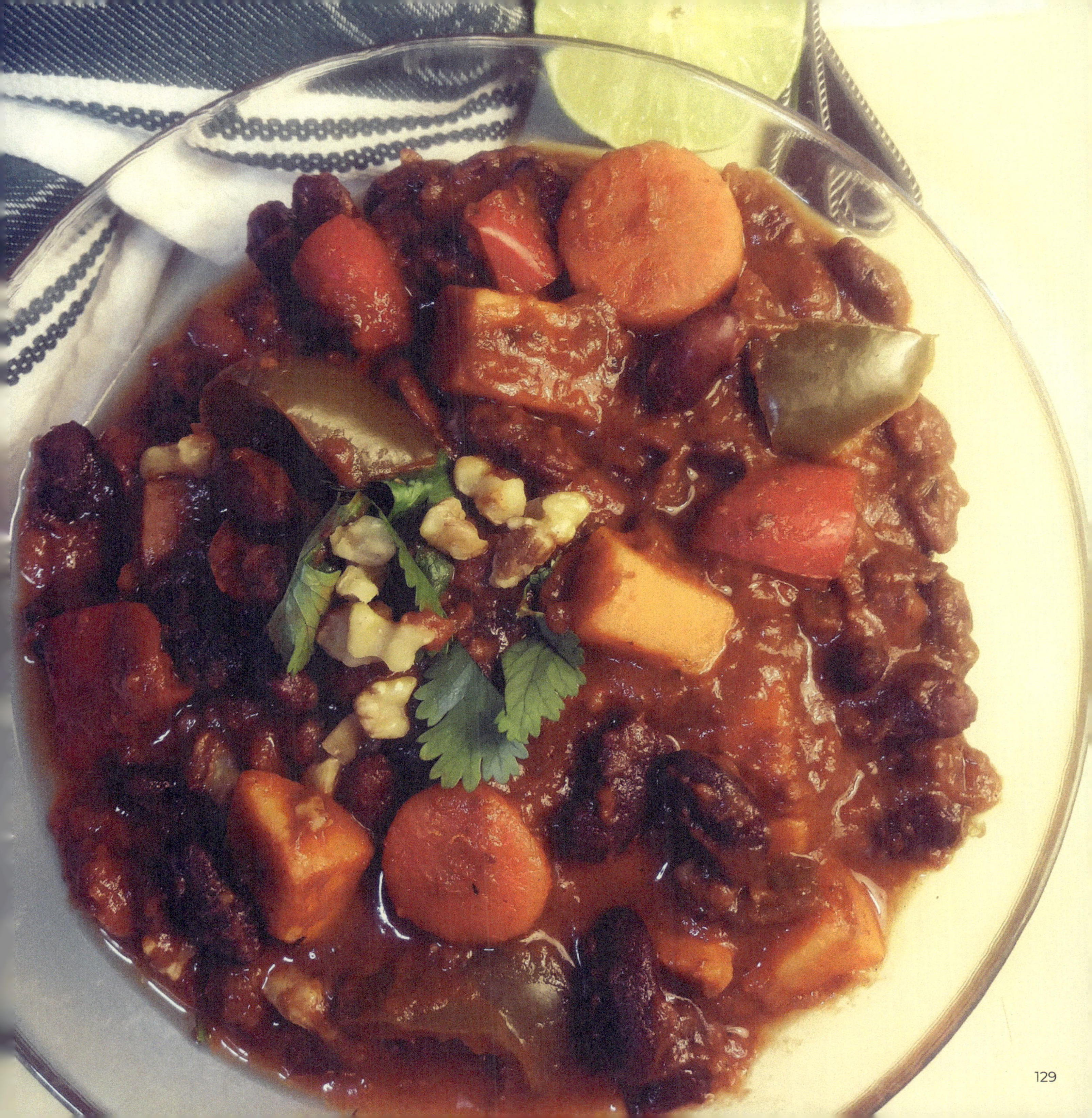

Winter Vegetables and Fruit

(partial listing)

Broccoli

Brussels sprouts

Cabbage

Cauliflower

Celeriac

Kabocha (winter) Squash

Parsnips

Rutabaga

Citrus fruits — Lemon, Lime, Orange, Tangerine

Pomegranate

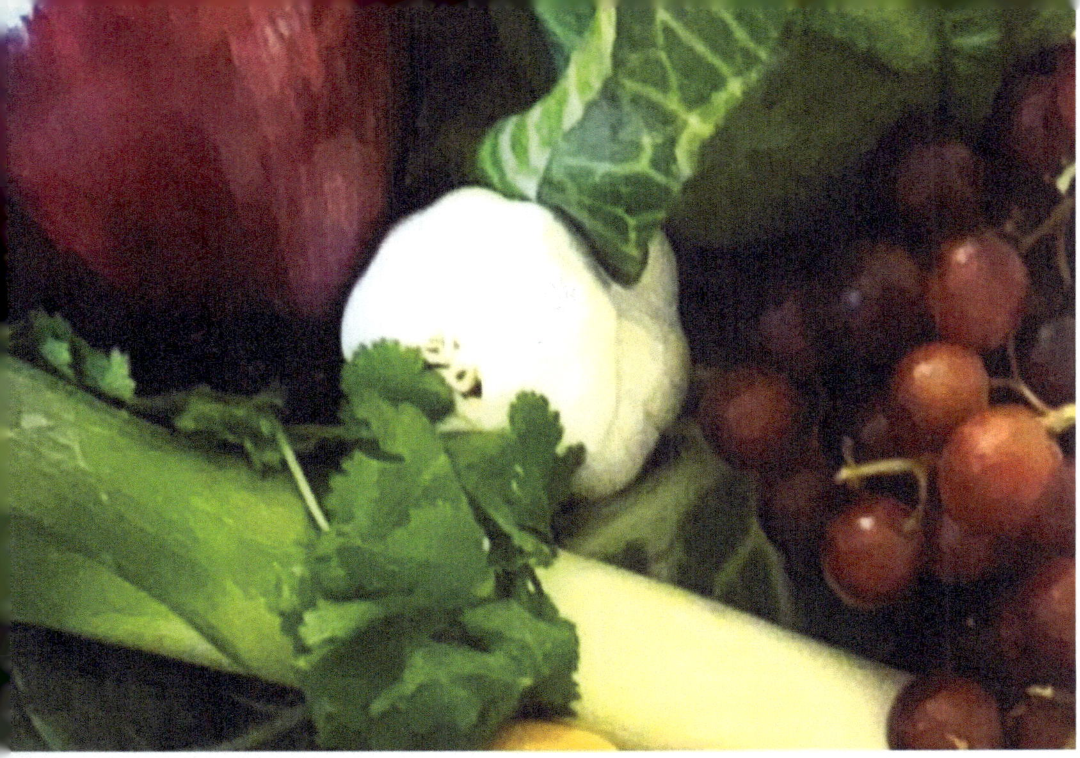

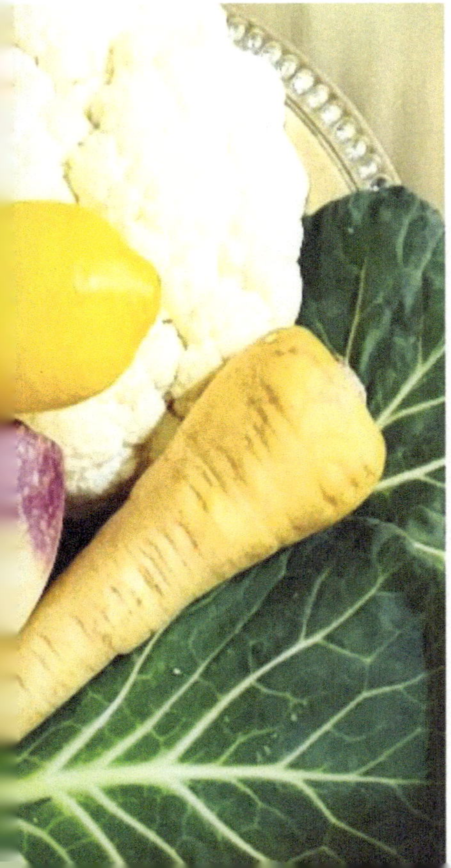

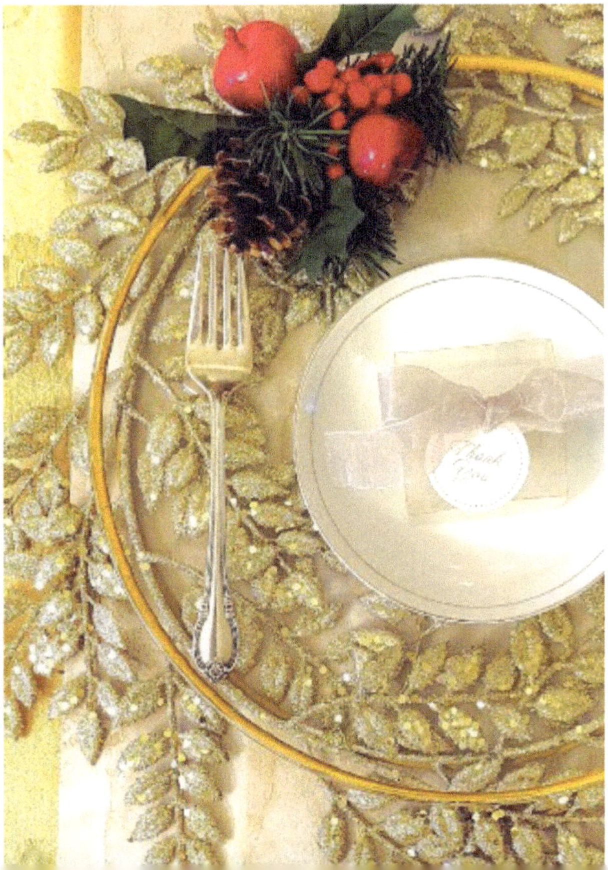

WINTER

DECEMBER, JANUARY + FEBRUARY

WINTER RECIPES

December is a month of holidays and celebration. Food always plays a major part at festive gatherings. Knowing that helps me adjust to the transition into cold weather. The secret is to hold onto those festive thoughts until March!

With shortened days and less time spent outdoors, winter is an excellent time for making relaxed meals. It's also a great time to appreciate slow-simmering hearty soups, stews, broths and "pot likkers." Our bodies need moisture, hydration, and nourishing food even more throughout the coldest season of the year.

Farmers and nature produce an array of hearty, nutrient-dense foods to celebrate the end-of-the-year season. Brussel sprouts, kale, leeks, broccoli rabe, and celery root grace markets along with the magnificent citrus varieties of the season: lemons, limes, oranges, blood oranges, tangerines, grapefruits, kumquats, and pomegranates all exemplify seasonal eating at its best. Legumes and grains balance out our plates.

Fruit and nut oils like olive oil, avocado oil, and almond oil are excellent in food preparation. These oils also can benefit us externally when applied to the skin for protection from the wind and cold of winter. Dried herbs and spices enhance the aroma and flavor of foods in the winter. Many of these herbs have medicinal properties that can boost the nutritional quality of our food as well as support our well-being.

Winter is a time to rest, reflect, retool, and prepare for the next season of our life and for the New Year.

Let's welcome winter!

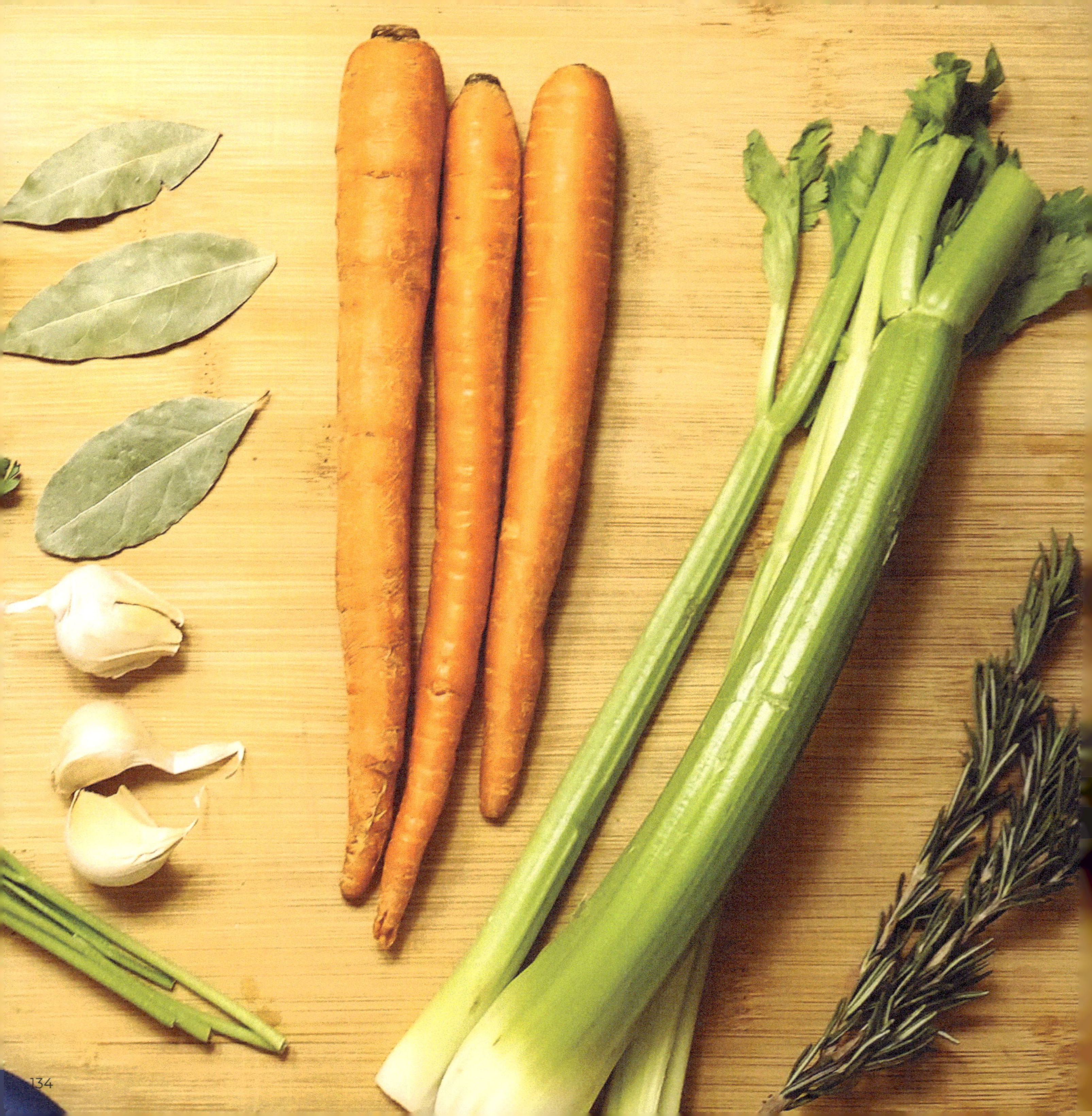

HEARTY VEGETABLE BROTH

I can remember purchasing broth maybe once or twice, but it didn't deliver what I needed, so I began making my own broth years ago and still do. The routine of making it is now part of my cooking—I just start with some basic aromatics and add seasonal vegetables as I like. Broth can be used in beans, stews, and also as a substitute for water in savory recipes. (Note: If these items are not regularly handy in your refrigerator, don't fret—just purchase broth or stock.)

INGREDIENTS:
5 cups water
3 ribs celery, chopped
3 carrots, chopped
1 large onion, chopped
2 cloves garlic
2 bay leaves
Handful of fresh parsley leaves

PREPARATION:
Add all ingredients to a large soup pot and gently simmer over medium-low heat for 35 minutes. Remove the bay leaves before serving.

Note: Good broth contains about:
50% onions
25% carrots
25% celery
...and parsley and bay leaves

Note: The following vegetables will turn the broth bitter:

Artichokes	Bell peppers	All members of the cabbage family
Cauliflower	Broccoli	Kale
Brussels sprouts	Kohlrabi	Turnips

Makes 12 ounces (1 ½ cups)

SPICY CAULIFLOWER

The Indian dish Aloo Gobi Masala was my inspiration for this dish. The first time I prepared the cauliflower, spices, and tomatoes only, I loved it. It has now become a quick go-to spicy dish for me. This version is a quick side dish and not as elaborate as the full Aloo Gobi. (Note: If you want a less spicy dish, omit the garam masala.)

INGREDIENTS:

1 tablespoon coconut oil
1 onion, coarsely chopped
2 cloves garlic, diced
One 28-ounce can of whole plum tomatoes (chopped)
1 cauliflower, cut into flowerets (approx. 4 cups)
1 teaspoon ground turmeric
1 teaspoon ground cumin
1 teaspoon ground ginger
¼ teaspoon red chili powder
½ teaspoon garam masala
Dash of cayenne pepper and sea salt

PREPARATION:

1. Warm the coconut oil in a medium-size soup pot over medium-low heat. Add the onion and garlic and sauté for 2 minutes. Stir in the tomatoes, cauliflower, and spices.
2. Cook for 15 minutes or until the vegetables are fork-tender. Pepper and salt to taste.

Makes 4 servings

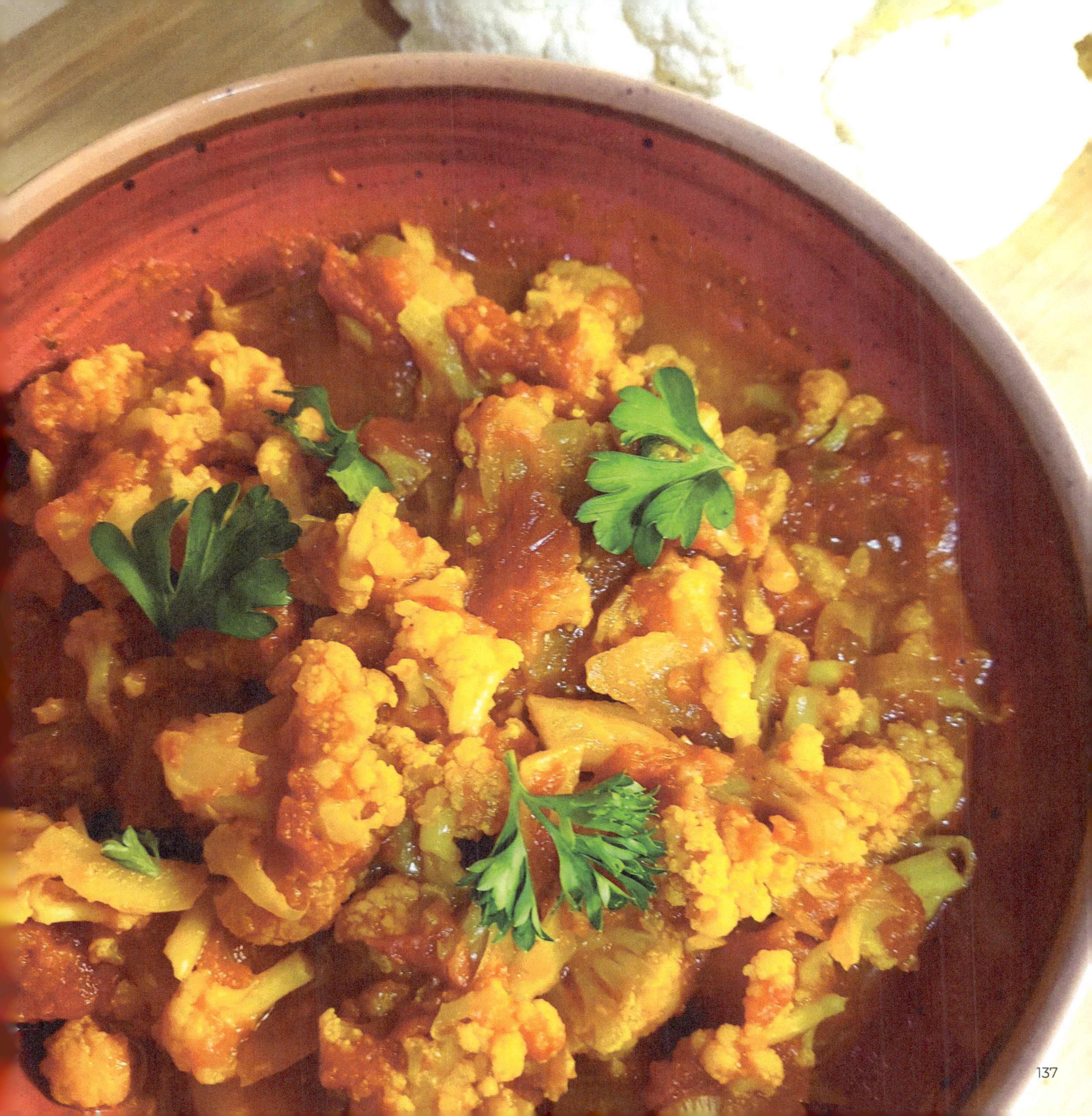

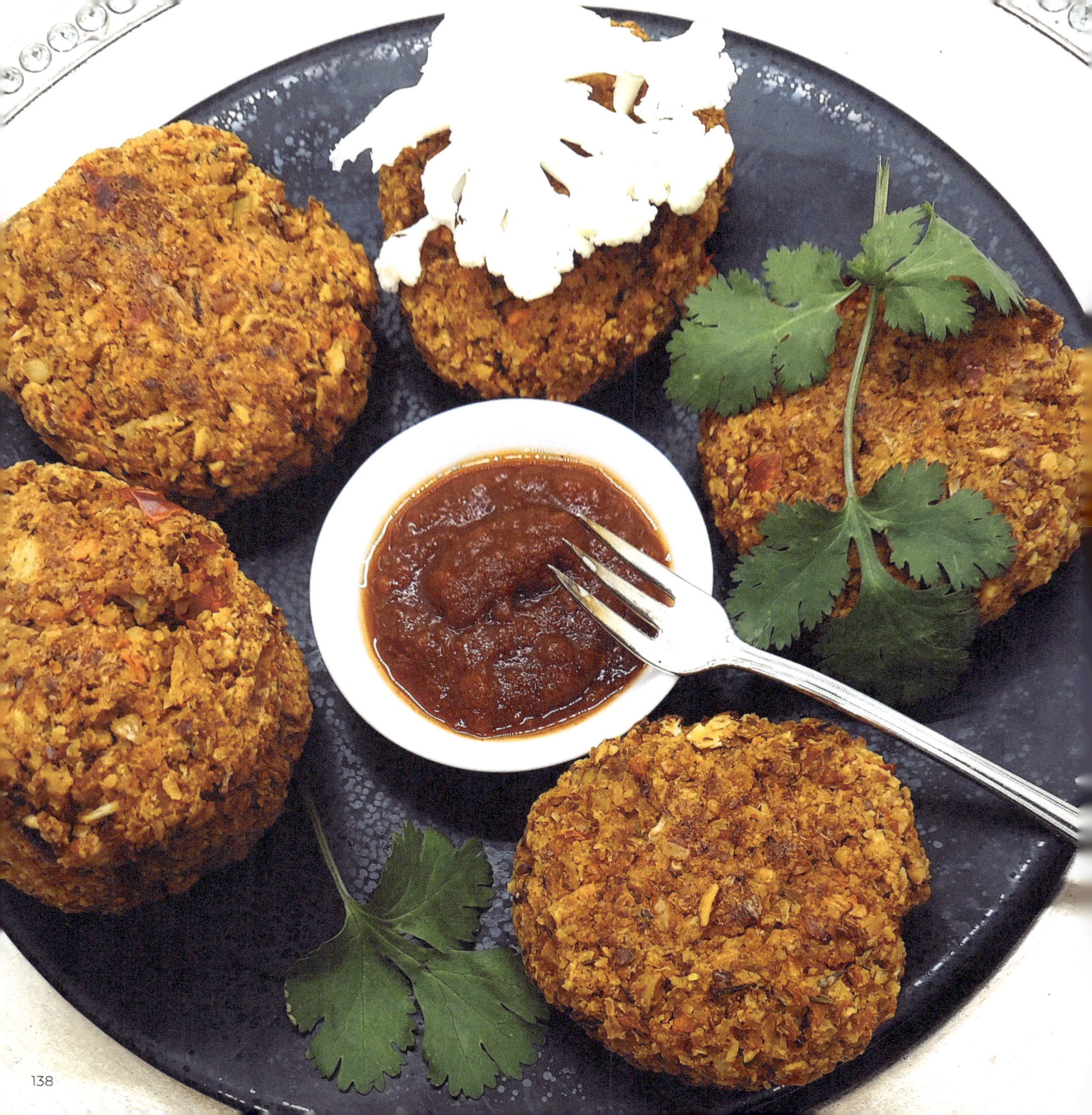

CAULIFLOWER - PARSNIP VEGGIE PATTIE

Cauliflower and parsnips make a great combination in this tasty veggie pattie, and the mixture is very pliable and easy to work with. Parsnips are full of vitamin C and potassium. I absolutely love this taste blend!

INGREDIENTS:

1 tablespoon ground flaxseeds
1 tablespoon coconut oil
1 small onion, diced (about ½ cup)
3 cloves garlic, minced
1 carrot, chopped
½ red bell pepper, diced
½ parsnip, grated (about 1 cup)
½ head of cauliflower, grated (about 2 cups)
1 teaspoon ground cumin
1 teaspoon ground coriander
1 teaspoon smoked paprika
½ teaspoon ground ginger
½ teaspoon dried thyme
Handful of fresh cilantro leaves, chopped
½ teaspoon Celtic sea salt
Dash of cayenne pepper
1 cup almonds, ground (almond meal can also be used)

PREPARATION: Preheat the oven to 350°F.

1. In a small bowl, mix the ground flaxseeds with 3 tablespoons of water. Let the mixture stand for 3 minutes to thicken.
2. Warm the oil in a large skillet over medium-low heat. Stir in the onion and garlic and cook for 2 minutes. Stir in the carrot, red pepper, and parsnip. Reduce heat and cook for 2 minutes. Cover and turn off the heat.
3. Place the cauliflower in a large bowl. Add the cooked vegetable mixture, flaxseed mixture, spices, thyme, cilantro, salt, and pepper. Mix well.
4. Add the ground almonds a little at a time. Knead with your hands, working the mixture until it's firm enough to form into patties.
5. Form into 6 patties. Place them on a baking sheet lined with parchment paper and bake for 15-20 minutes on each side.

Makes 6 patties

BLACK-EYED PEAS & COLLARD GREENS

Protein-rich black-eyed peas blend so well with the "queen of greens," collards! The only thing needed to enhance this wonderful dish is a cornbread muffin. Note: I do not soak black eyed peas overnight, I rinse them well, and cover with water just as I am preparing to cook.

INGREDIENTS:

2 cups dried black-eyed peas, sorted and rinsed
1 tablespoon coconut oil
1 onion, diced
3 cloves garlic, minced
2 ribs celery, diced
1 large carrot, diced
2 bay leaves
1 teaspoon smoked paprika
2 tablespoons tomato paste
Dash of cayenne pepper
½ teaspoon Celtic sea salt
6 collard leaves

PREPARATION:

1. In a large soup pot over low heat, add the coconut oil, onion, garlic, celery, and carrot and sauté for 2 minutes.

2. Add the black-eyed peas, 5 cups of water, and the bay leaves. Increase heat to medium and add the paprika, tomato paste, cayenne pepper, and salt. Bring it to a boil, then reduce heat to a simmer and cook for 10 minutes.

3. While the peas are cooking, stack the collard leaves, roll them into cylinders, and cut them into ribbons. (This is called a chiffonade cut.) Then chop the collards cross-wise and stir them into the peas adding additional water if the simmering liquid gets low.

4. Cook, covered, for 20 minutes. The soup is done when the peas and collards are fully cooked and tender to the touch of a fork. Remove the bay leaves before serving.

Makes 4 to 6 servings

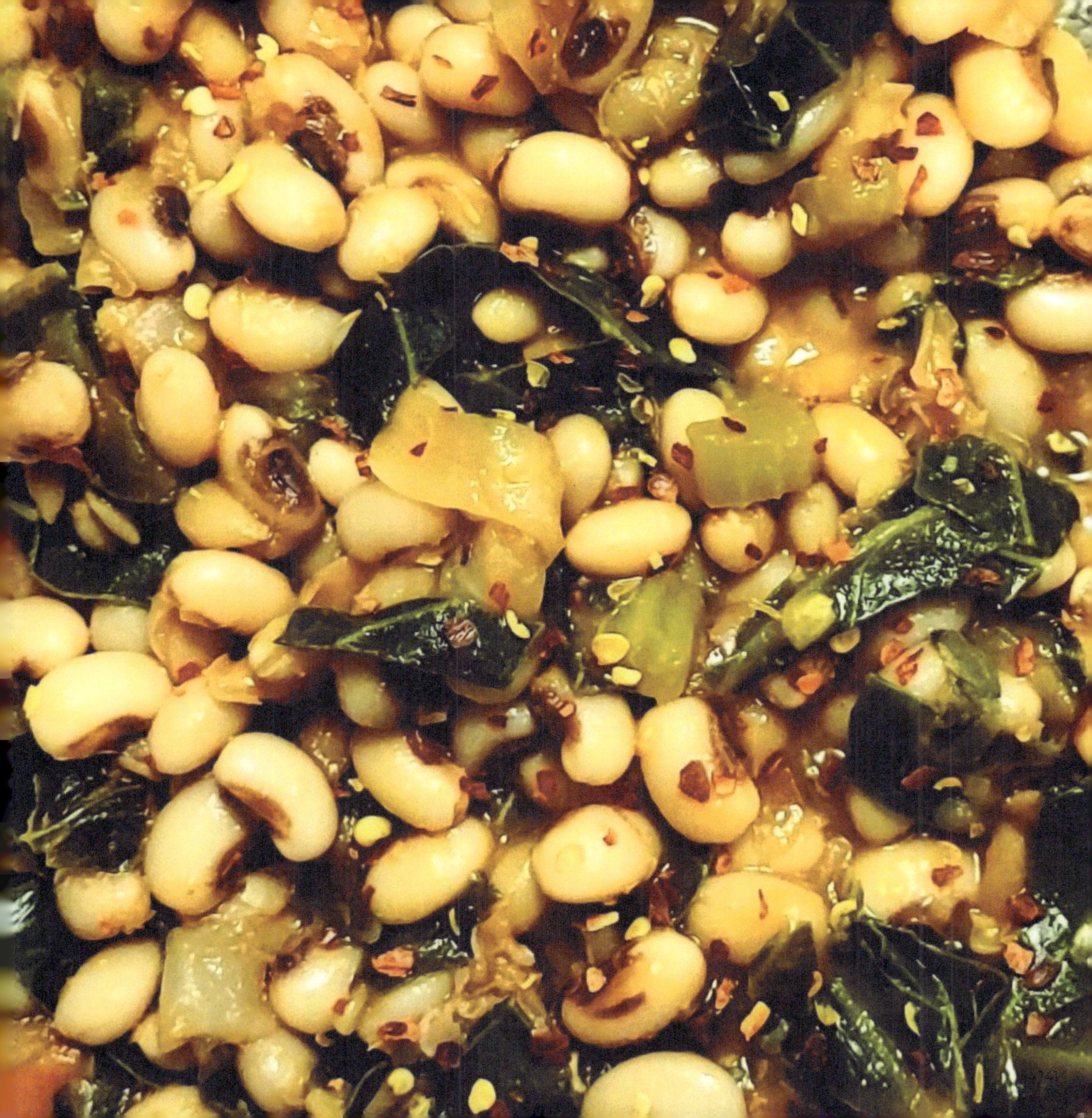

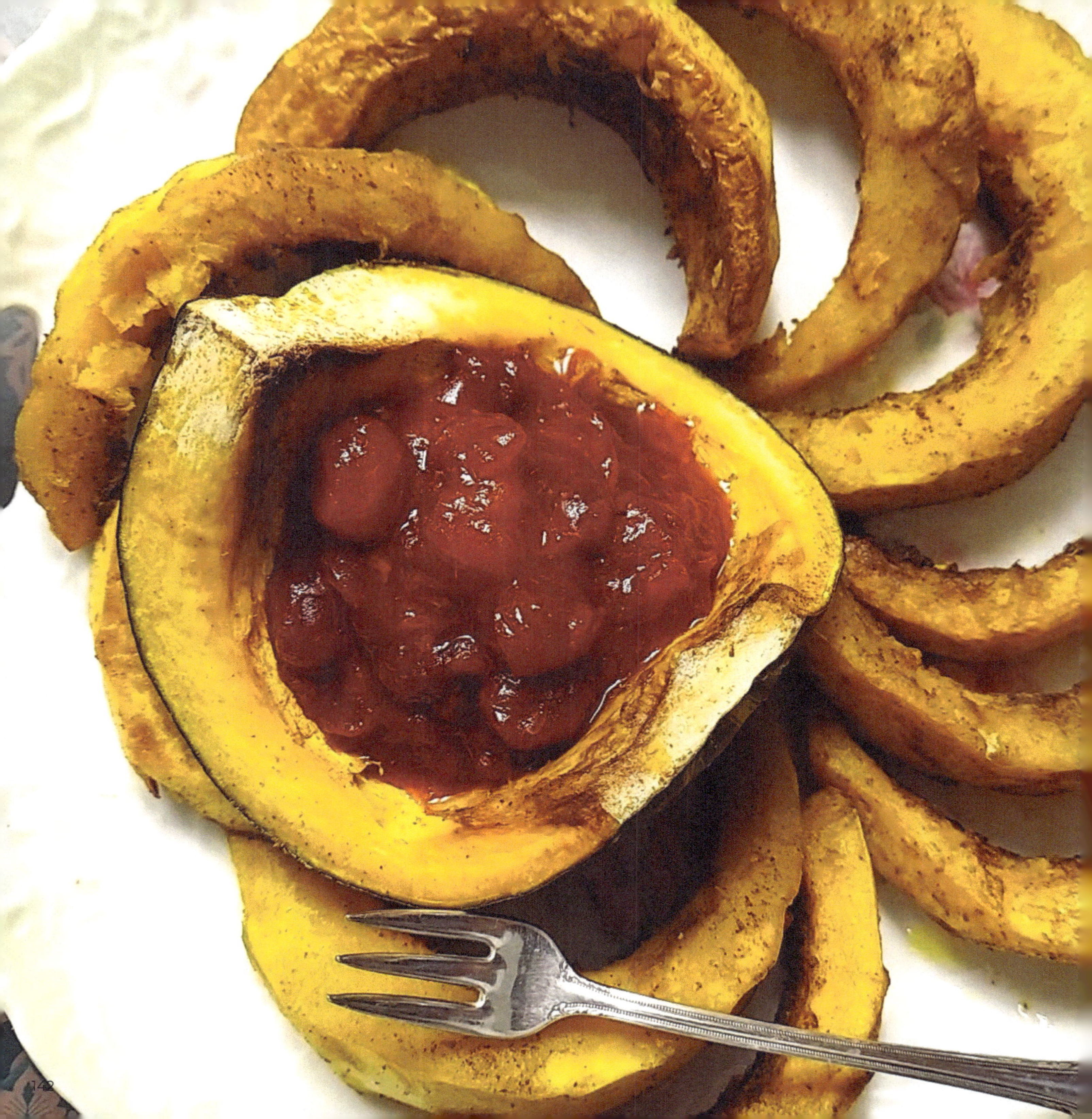

ROASTED KABOCHA SQUASH

Kabocha squash belongs to the winter squash family. This hard-shelled winter squash has more flavor and texture than a sweet potato. Also known as "Japanese pumpkin," it is an excellent source of beta-carotene, iron, copper, and magnesium.

INGREDIENTS:
1 small or medium kabocha squash or buttercup squash
¼ teaspoon ground nutmeg
¼ teaspoon ground cinnamon
½ teaspoon ground cumin
¼ teaspoon cayenne pepper
½ teaspoon Celtic sea salt
1 tablespoon olive oil

PREPARATION: Preheat oven to 400°F. Line a baking sheet with parchment paper.

1. Cut the squash in half and remove the seeds. Cut each half into equal wedges and peel to remove the outer shell. Place the squash slices in a large resealable bag.

2. Blend the spices and salt in a small bowl, then add the spices to the squash slices in the bag and shake well to coat.

3. Spread the coated squash slices out on the baking sheet and drizzle with olive oil. Roast in the oven until soft when pierced with a fork, approximately 15-20 minutes.

Makes 4 servings

MOROCCAN CHICKPEA STEW

Here, we have high-protein, high-fiber chickpeas blended with tomatoes, aromatic spices, caramelized red onion, dried apricots, lemon, and fresh greens in a dish that will warm your spirit.

INGREDIENTS:

¼ cup olive oil
3 large cloves garlic, halved
1 large red onion, sliced thinly
½ cup dried apricots (unsulphured), chopped
2 tablespoons garam masala
1 teaspoon Celtic sea salt
¾ teaspoon black pepper
1/4 teaspoon crushed red pepper
½ teaspoon of ground cinnamon
2 teaspoons fresh lemon juice
3½ cups cooked chickpeas or two 15-ounce cans chickpeas, rinsed and drained
One 28-ounce can diced tomatoes
4 cups escarole or curly spinach, chopped
1 cup loosely packed cilantro leaves
¼ cup loosely packed fresh mint leaves, chopped
Optional: Cooked brown rice for serving

PREPARATION:

1. In a large skillet over medium heat, warm the olive oil, add garlic cloves for 1 minute, then turn off heat (so not to burn) and remove garlic.

2. To the warm skillet, add the onions, apricots, garam masala, salt, black and red pepper, and cinnamon. Sauté for 8 minutes over low heat, stirring occasionally. Add ½ cup water, lemon juice, chickpeas, and the tomatoes. Bring to a boil, then reduce the heat to low and simmer for 7 minutes, occasionally stirring.

3. Stir in the escarole or spinach and simmer until the greens have wilted, about 5 minutes.

4. Remove from heat, stir in cilantro leaves and mint leaves. Serve as is or over brown rice.

Makes 4 to 6 servings

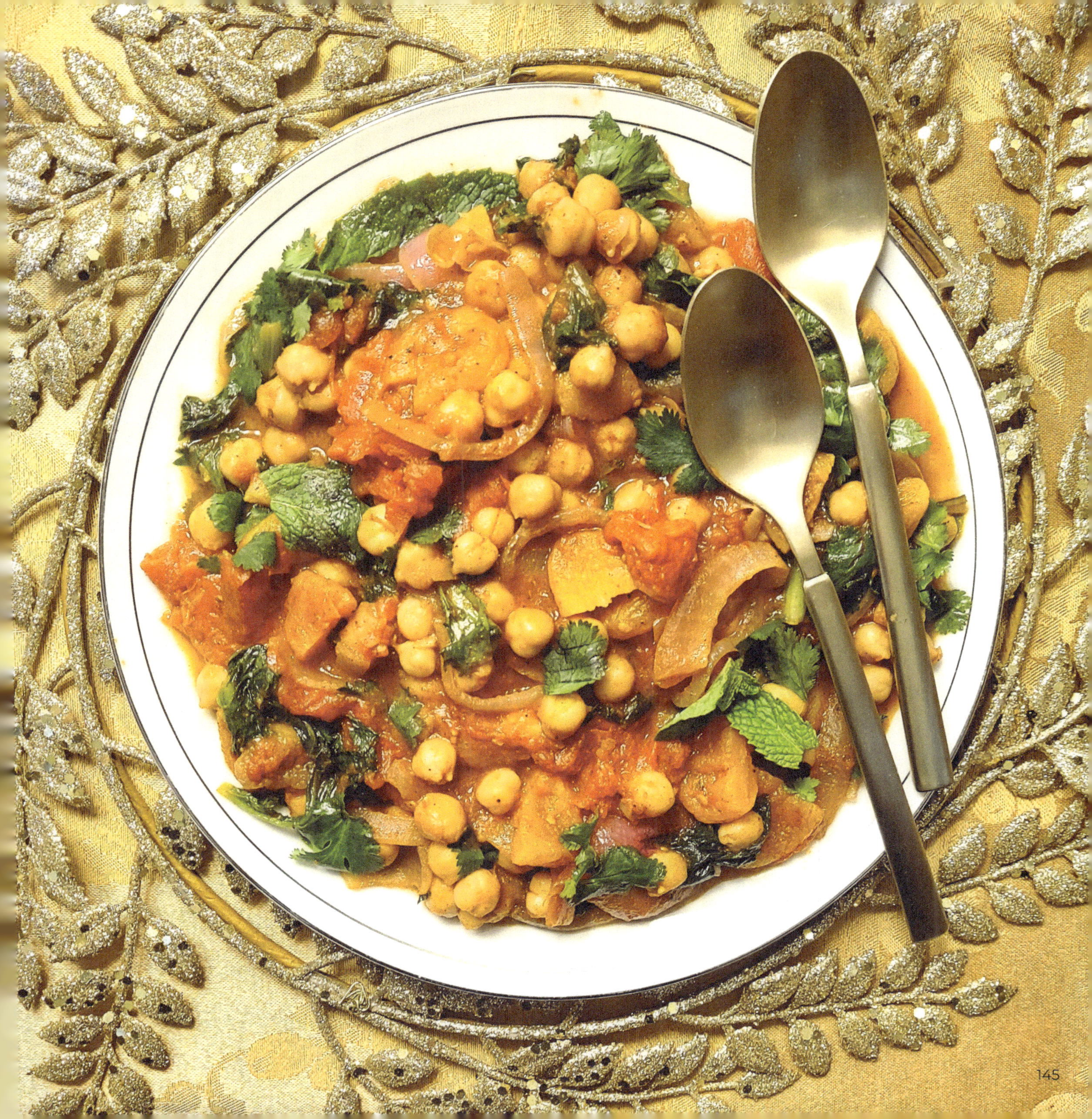

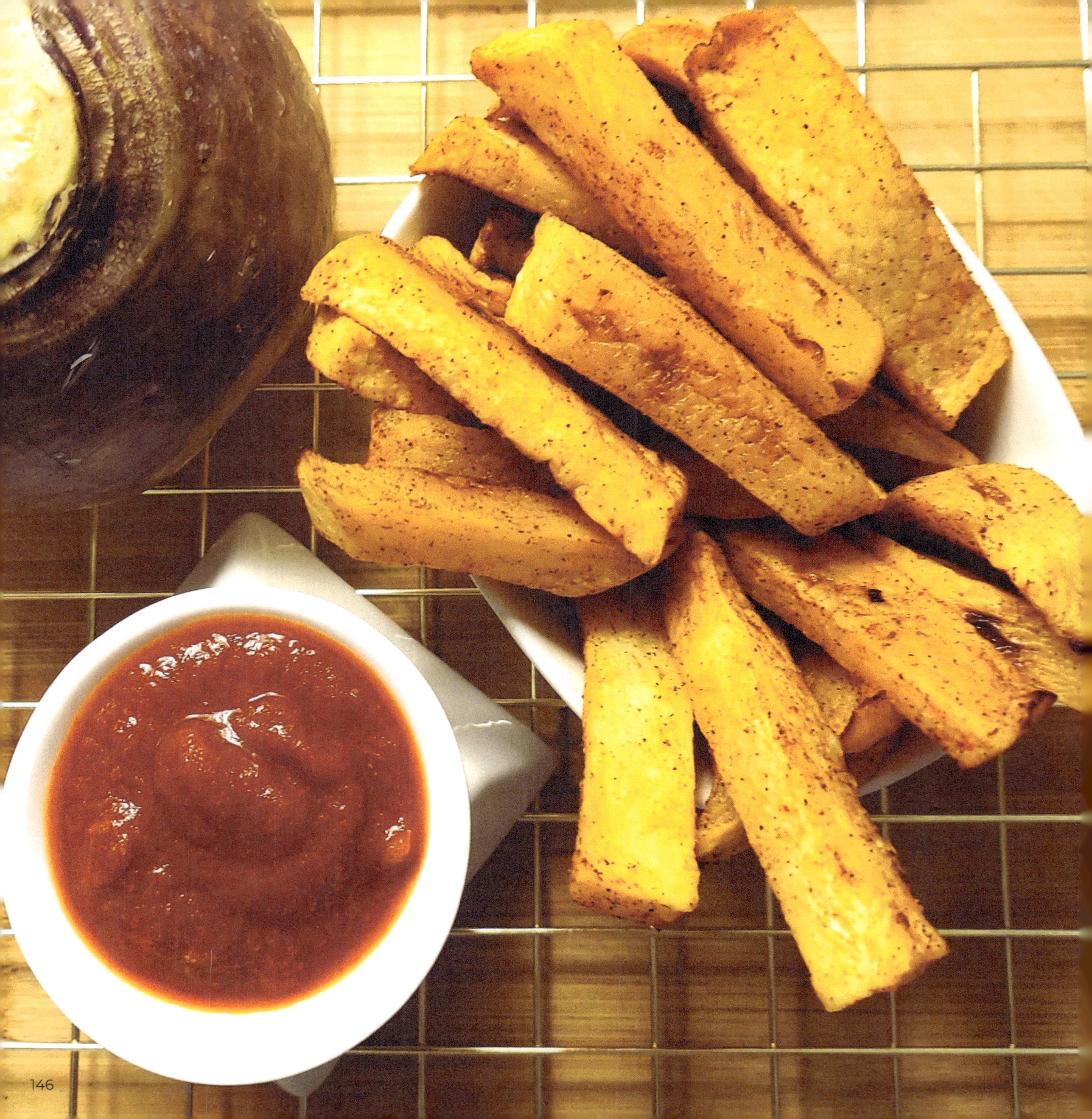

OVEN-ROASTED RUTABAGA WEDGES

This root vegetable is rich in potassium, calcium, and vitamin C, slightly bitter but sweeter than a turnip. Rutabagas at the Farmer's market will not be waxed and may have their greens attached. Roasted rutabagas are a healthy alternative to roasted potatoes. They can also be simmered in stews and soups.

INGREDIENTS:
1 medium rutabaga
1 teaspoon coconut oil (melted)
½ teaspoon ground cinnamon
Pinch of cayenne pepper
¼ teaspoon Celtic sea salt

PREPARATION: Preheat oven to 400° F.

1. Peel the rutabaga and cut it into wedges. Toss with coconut oil and sprinkle with cinnamon, pepper, and salt.
2. Arrange on a parchment paper lined baking pan and roast for 15 minutes or until tender when pierced with a fork. Serve with your favorite condiment.

Makes 2-3 servings

EINKORN (WHEAT BERRY) BOWL

Einkorn is an ancient grain that is being revived. Ancient grains are a group of grains and pseudo cereals (seeds that are consumed like grains) that have remained mostly unchanged for thousands of years. Einkorn has a nutty flavor and a rich texture, its high protein and beta-carotene content "sealed the deal with me," as the saying goes. This is another grain you can cook in quantity and use in a stir-fry, stew, or hearty salad.

INGREDIENTS:

1 cup einkorn (wheat berries or farro can be a substitute)
1 medium sweet potato, peeled and cut into small chunks
2 teaspoons olive oil, divided
½ teaspoon ground cinnamon
½ teaspoon smoked paprika
½ of a medium onion, chopped (about ½ cup)
2 cloves garlic, minced
8 ounces button mushrooms, sliced
1 teaspoon ground cumin
1 teaspoon ground ginger
1 teaspoon ground turmeric
½ teaspoon black pepper

PREPARATION:

1. In a medium-size saucepan, add 1 cup of einkorn to 3 cups of water. Bring to a boil, then lower heat to a simmer and cook for 40 minutes covered or until all of the water has been absorbed into the grain.

2. In a bowl, toss the sweet potatoes with 1 teaspoon of oil. Dust with the cinnamon, paprika, and cayenne. Toss the potatoes well to coat them. Place on a baking pan lined with parchment paper and bake for approximately 10 minutes.

3. In a medium-size skillet over low heat, add the remaining oil and the onion, garlic, and mushrooms. Cover and allow mushrooms to sweat for 3 minutes. Uncover and stir in the spices and pepper.

4. Add the cooked einkorn to a bowl and stir in the mushroom mixture and the potatoes. Serve while hot.

Makes 4 servings

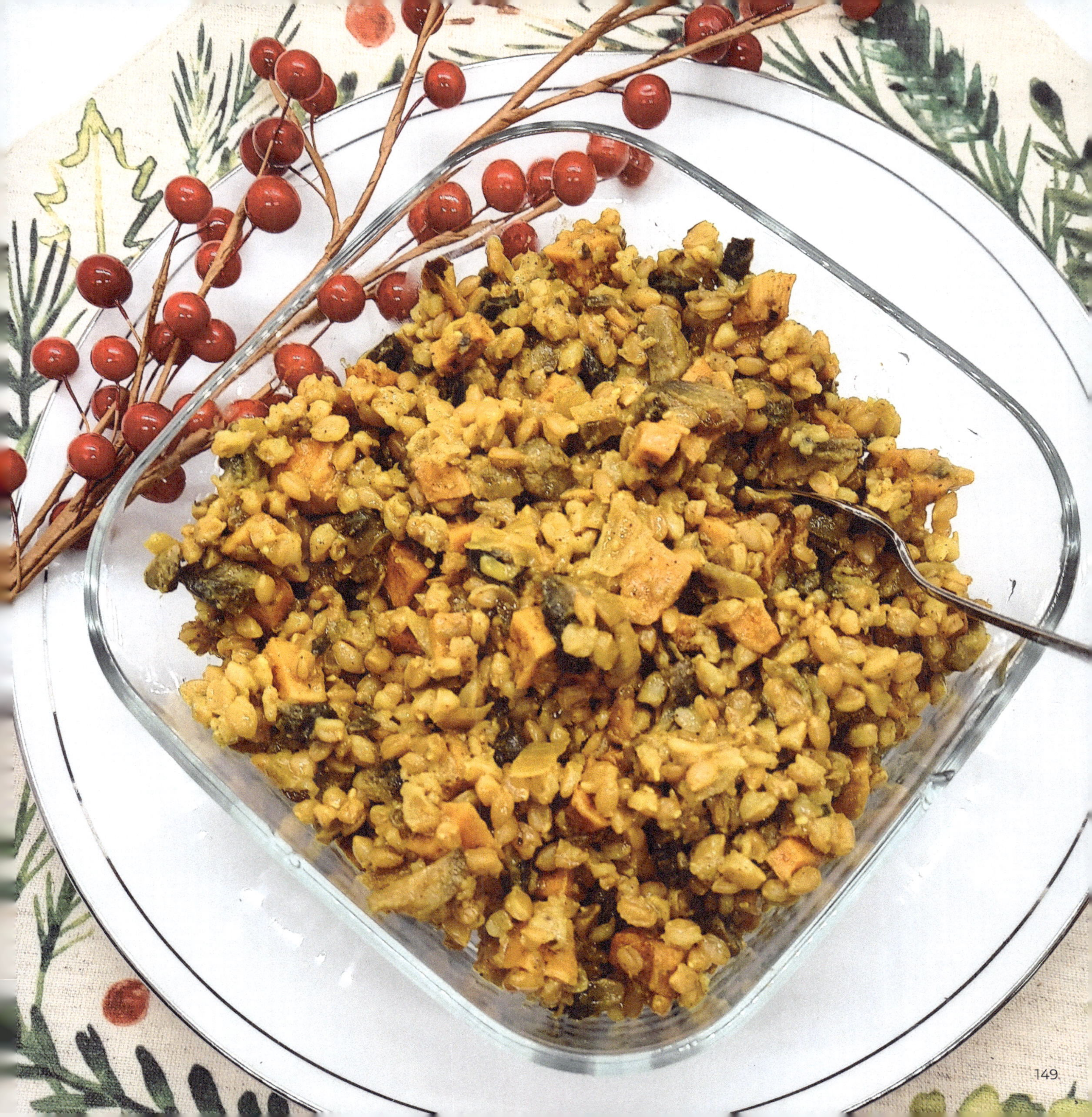

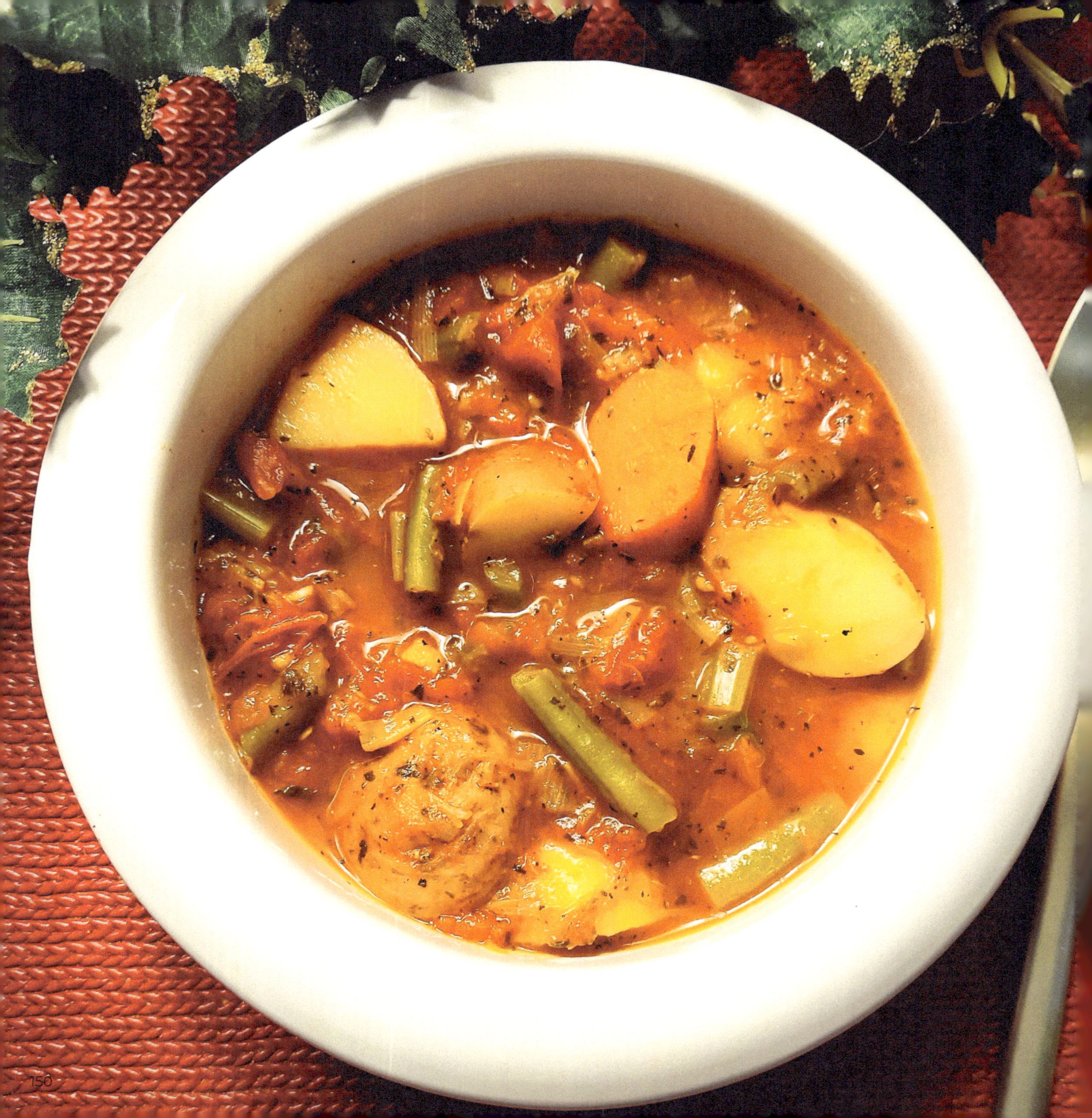

SAVORY WINTER VEGGIE SOUP

Nothing warms the body like a hearty bowl of soup on a wintry January day! This soup has character and a little sass with a flavorful, savory taste.

INGREDIENTS:

3½ cups vegetable broth, divided
1 leek, white part only, rinse thoroughly sliced thin
1 rib celery, chopped
3 cloves garlic, diced
2 carrots, sliced on the diagonal
2 teaspoons dried basil
1 teaspoon dried thyme
1 teaspoon smoked paprika
½ teaspoon pepper
One 28-ounce can of plum tomatoes,
8 ounces green beans, rinsed and cut into bite-size pieces
8 ounces of multicolored petite potatoes, sliced in halves

PREPARATION:

1. Warm ½ cup of the vegetable broth in a large soup pot over medium-low heat. Add the leek, celery, garlic, and carrots and simmer for 3 minutes.
2. Add the herbs, smoked paprika, pepper, tomatoes, and remaining broth and cook for 10 minutes.
3. Add the green beans and potatoes and cook until they're tender to the touch of the fork, approximately 15 minutes.

Makes 4 servings

STEWED CABBAGE WITH PEPPERS

Cabbage is a cruciferous vegetable, studies consistently show that diets high in cruciferous vegetables are associated with lower incidents of cancer. Cabbage is economical and one of the most nutritious vegetables we can eat.

INGREDIENTS:

1 tablespoon coconut oil
1 medium onion, chopped
1 clove garlic, diced
1 carrot, sliced into coins
1 head cabbage, sliced thinly
2 tablespoons tomato paste
2 teaspoons smoked paprika
2 teaspoons ground ginger
½ teaspoon sea salt
Dash cayenne pepper
1 bell pepper, coarsely chopped

PREPARATION:

1. In a large soup pot over medium-low heat, warm the coconut oil. Add the onion, garlic, and carrot and sauté for 2 minutes. Add the cabbage, a cup of water and cook for about 3 minutes, stirring until the cabbage begins to wilt.
2. Stir in the tomato paste, spices, salt, and pepper. Add 3 cups of water to cover the vegetables. Cook over medium-low heat for 20 minutes. Add the bell peppers and cook until peppers are tender to the touch of a fork, approximately 10 minutes.

Makes 4 to 6 servings

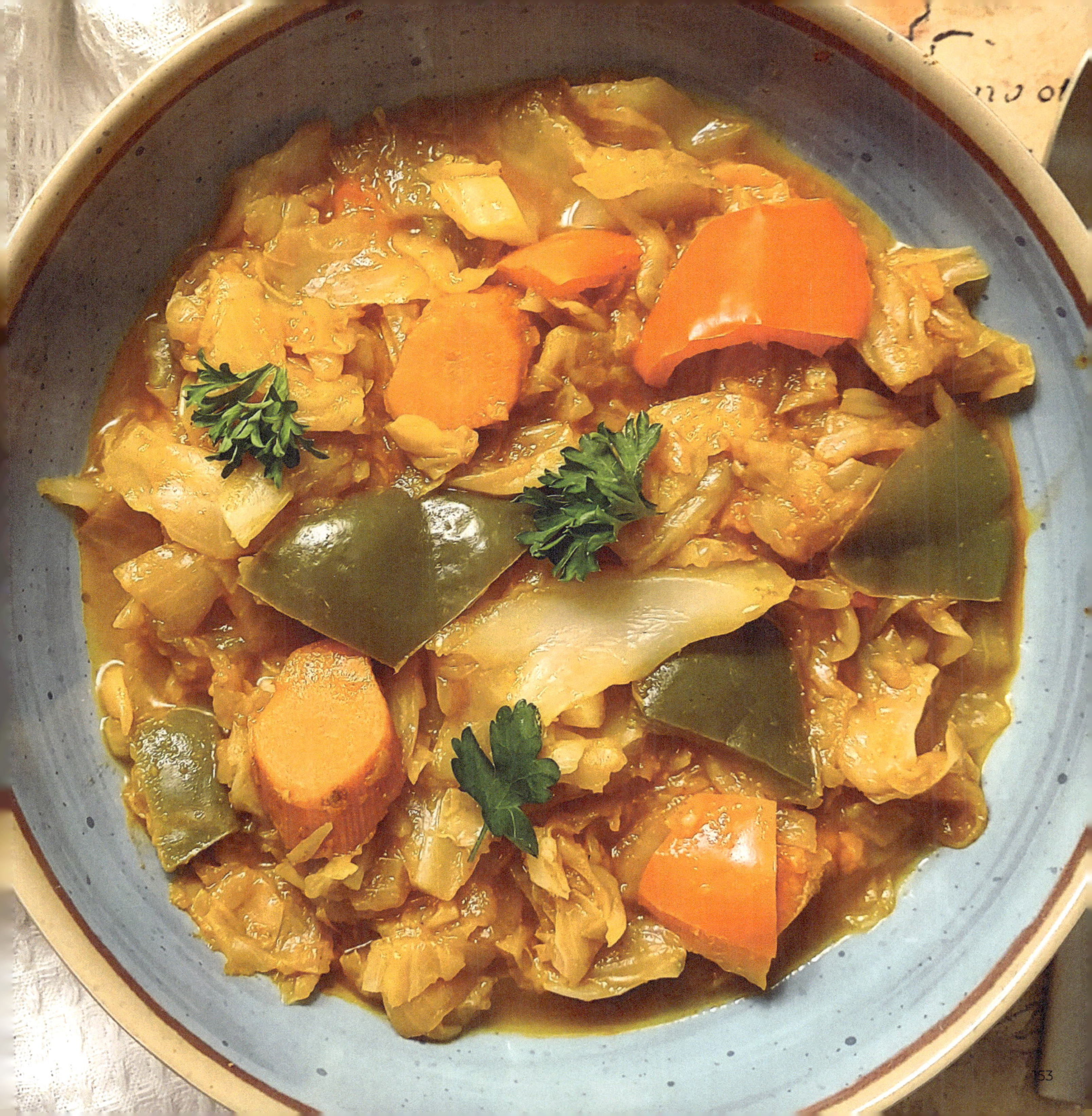

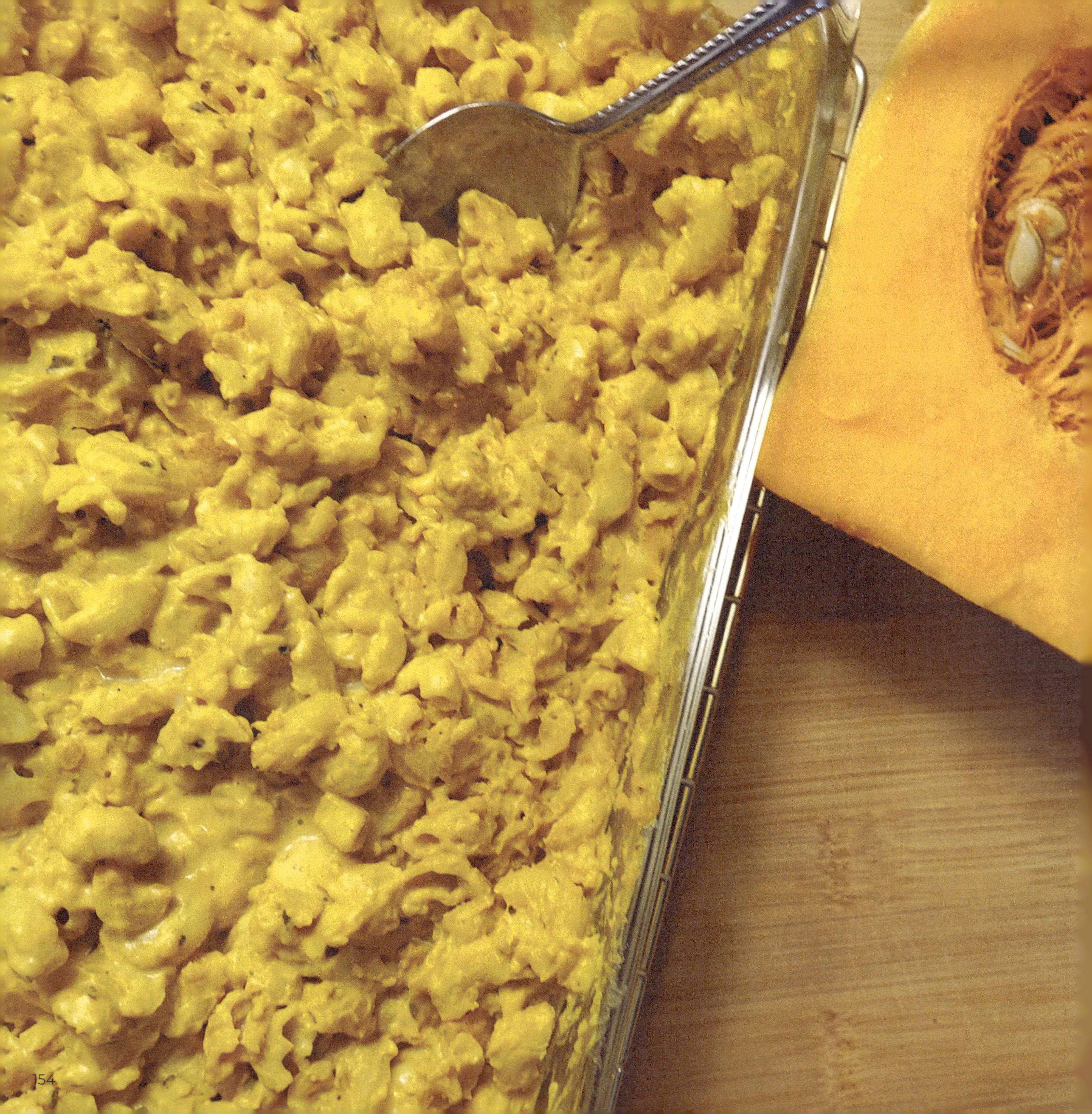

MAC AND BUTTERNUT CHEESE

This is pure comfort food and with plants, your arteries are not at risk. Butternut squash and cashews make this smooth cream sauce. Enjoy the sauce also as a dip, a sauce, or an ingredient. This is made with NO plant-based cheese

INGREDIENTS:

2 cups of butternut squash, peeled in cubes
1- 8-ounce box chickpea elbow pasta
1 teaspoon olive oil
1 cup of raw cashews,
3 tablespoons nutritional yeast
2 cloves of garlic, chopped
2 tablespoons whole grain mustard (see recipe page. 196)
2 tablespoons lemon juice
1 can (13.5 oz) coconut milk (almond milk can be used)
2 teaspoons smoked paprika
2 teaspoons turmeric
½ teaspoon onion powder
½ teaspoon Celtic Sea salt (optional)

PREPARATION: Preheat oven to 375°F; oil casserole or baking pan (9 x 11)

1. Cover cashews with water, allow to sit for ½ hour, drain and set aside
2. Place squash cubes in a bowl, sprinkle olive oil and toss to coat well. Pour onto a parchment paper lined baking pan, roast 20 minutes or until tender.
3. Prepare the pasta according to box instruction. Add to rapid boiling water, stir immediately. Cook 8 minutes, drain. Rinse well under warm water.
4. Add squash, cashews, nutritional yeast, garlic, mustard, lemon juice, milk, paprika, turmeric, onion powder to a high speed blender and blend until smooth.
5. Taste sauce and add additional seasonings to your taste. Oil casserole or baking pan. Add pasta, mix in butternut-cashew sauce. Pop in oven Bake 25-30 minutes.

Leftover butternut cheese sauce will last 4-5 days refrigerated in an air-tight container.

Makes 32 ounces

ROASTED BROCCOLI WITH VEGAN CHEESE SAUCE

Broccoli falls in the brassica family of cruciferous vegetables. They include: broccoli, kale, bok choy, mustard greens, cauliflower, cabbage, arugula, watercress and turnips. Many studies show that the higher the intake of these foods, the lower the risk of cancer. This yummy cheese sauce is made of potatoes and carrots.

INGREDIENTS:

1 bunch of broccoli, florets only (about 3.5 cups)
1 tablespoon olive oil
2 clove garlic, sliced
1 teaspoon smoked paprika
Sprinkle of pepper
Optional: additional root veggies can be added

Cheese Sauce: Makes 1 cup
1 large potato, cut into chunks
2 carrots, cut into chunks
¾ cup of non-diary milk
½ lemon, juiced
¾ teaspoon onion powder
¾ teaspoon garlic powder
¾ teaspoon smoked paprika
2 tablespoons Whole grain mustard (see page 196)
Celtic sea salt and pepper, as you like
1 tablespoon olive oil

PREPARATION: Pre-heat oven to 425° F.

1. Place broccoli florets in bowl, toss with olive oil, season with smoked paprika, pepper and sprinkle garlic slices. Transfer broccoli to a baking sheet lined with parchment paper.

2. Roast in pre-heated oven until the broccoli is tender and lightly browned. About 15-20 minutes.

Prepare Cheese Sauce:

3. Place potatoes and carrots in small pot with 3 cups of water and boil until tender to the touch of a fork. Drain and transfer to a high-speed blender. Add milk, lemon juice, onion powder and garlic powder, smoked paprika, mustard, salt, pepper and olive oil - blend for one minute. Taste and make adjustments if needed.

4. Once broccoli is tender to the touch of a fork, serve with the dairy free cheese sauce.

Makes 4 servings

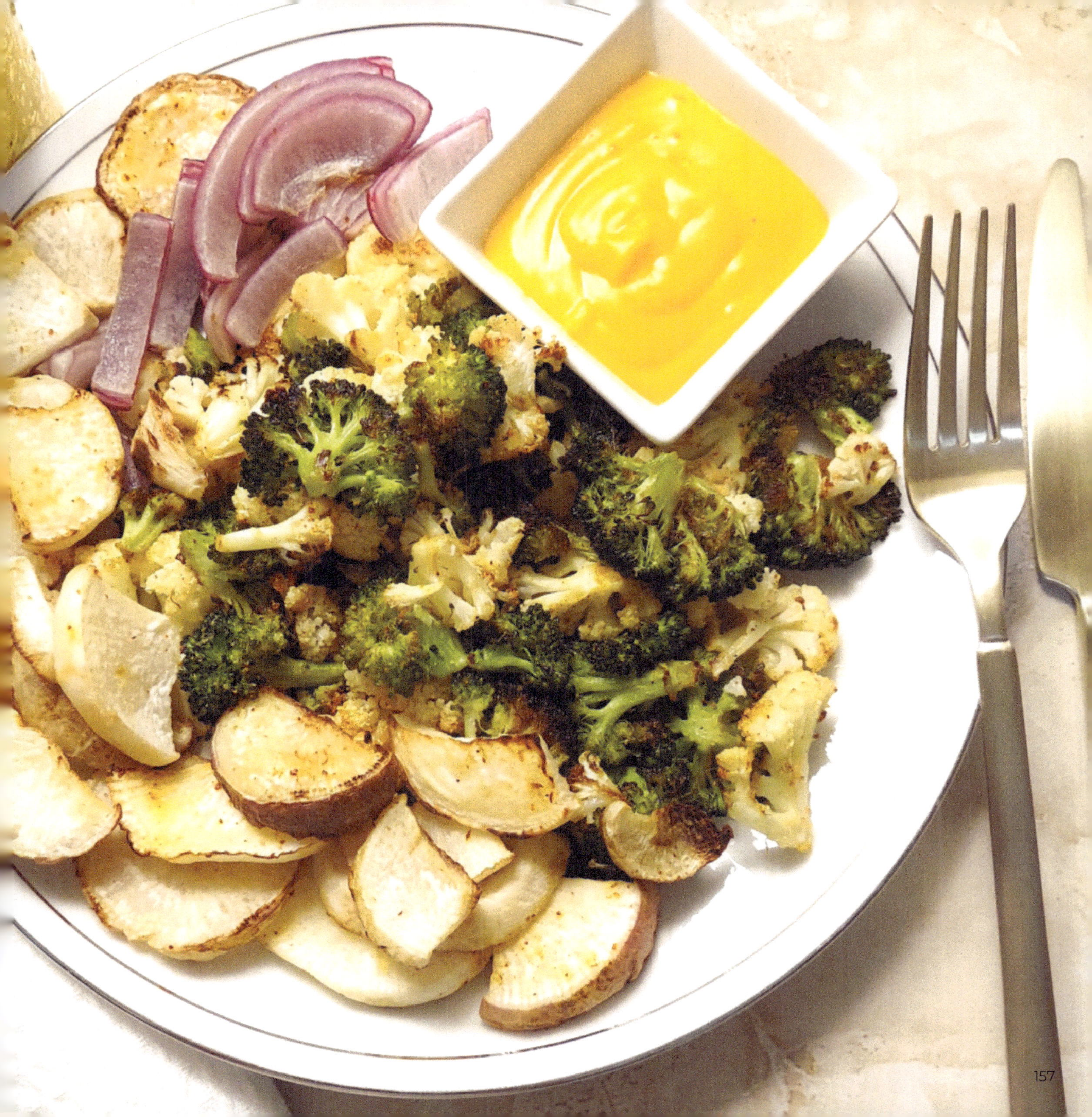

Breakfast Vegetables and Fruit

(partial listing)

Bell Pepper
Carrots
Kale
Mushroom
Onion
Potatoes (Red, Sweet, Yukon gold)
Spinach

Apple
Apricot
Avocado
Banana
Blackberry
Blueberry
Cranberry
Kiwi
Lemon, Lime
Pomegranate
Strawberry

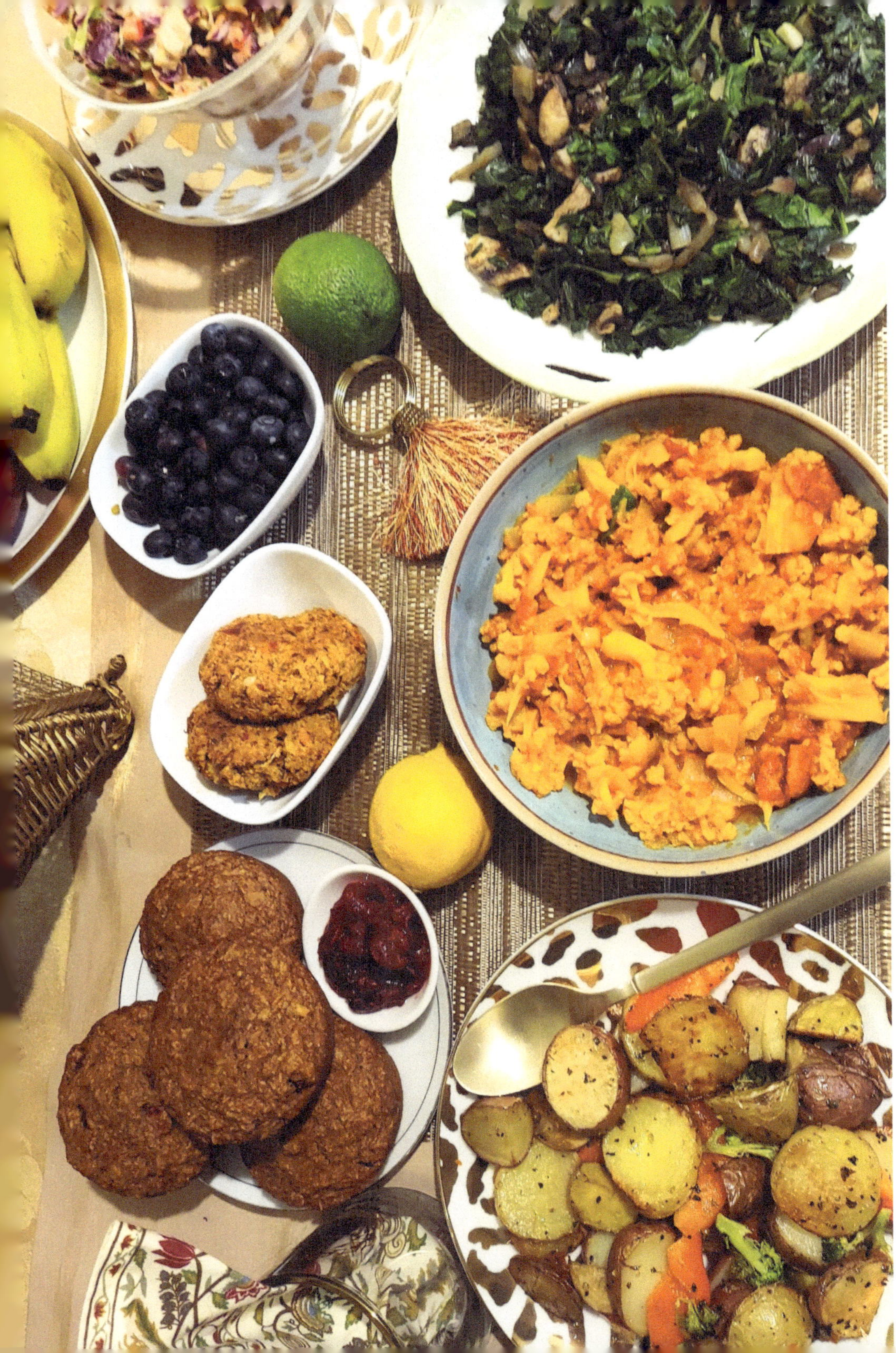

BREAKFAST

BREAKFAST RECIPES

Breakfast is the first meal of the day. When shifting from the Standard American Diet (SAD) to healthier food choices, the breakfast table includes new tastes. Here are some quick, healthy morning (or anytime) meal options:

1. Breakfast bowls: When time in the morning is at a premium, enjoy a Chia Seed-Fruit cup, a bowl of Crunchy Granola with fruit, or a hearty bowl of oatmeal.

2. Morning smoothies: Quick and nutrient packed. My personal go-to favorites are Red Russian Kale Smoothie or a Morning Berry Smoothie.

3. Breakfast comfort food: When there is time. Feast on a Potato - Veggie Skillet or Vegan Buttermilk Pancakes with Blueberry Compote.

4. Hot drink alternatives: Enjoy a delicious Roasted Chicory Dandelion Root sip, or Cacao Hot Chocolate w/whipped cream.

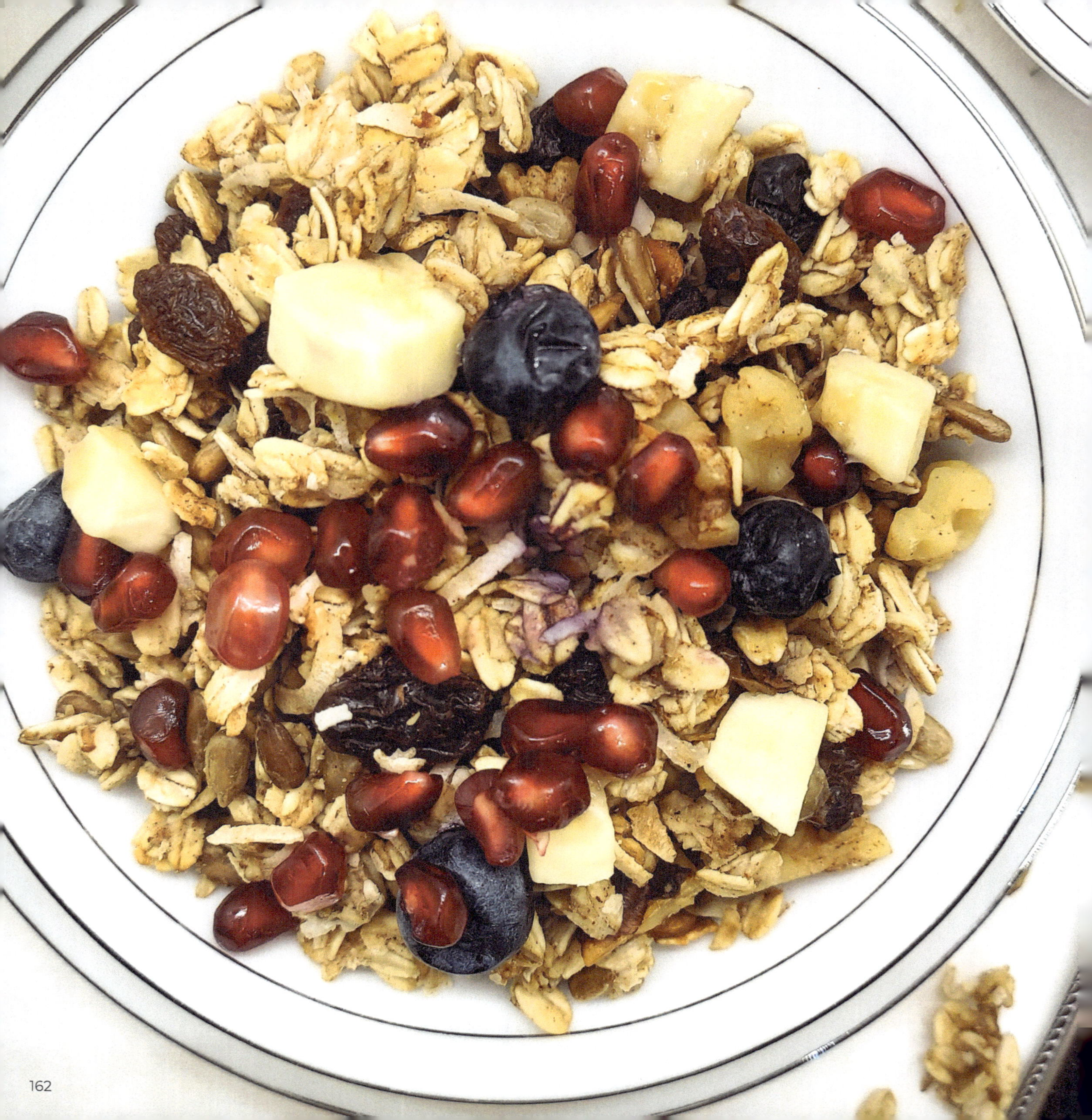

HEALTHY CRUNCHY GRANOLA

Making this quick and easy granola gives you control over the sugar, salt, and other ingredients. Use this recipe as a template and include your selection of ingredients.

INGREDIENTS:
2 cups rolled oats
3/4 cup raw walnuts, chopped
1/2 cup raw sunflower seeds
1/2 teaspoon ground cinnamon
Pinch of nutmeg
1 ripe large banana,
½ cup non-dairy milk
1 tablespoon coconut oil
1 teaspoon vanilla extract
1 tablespoon - maple syrup
½ cup raisins (or dried fruit of your choice)
Optional: Ground flax seeds to sprinkle

PREPARATION: Pre-heat oven to 250°F.

1. In a large mixing bowl, combine the oats, nuts, seeds, cinnamon.
2. In a small bowl, mash the banana, add milk, oil, vanilla, and maple syrup. Pour the liquid ingredients into the dry mixture and mix well.
3. Spread the mixture out on a rimmed baking sheet and bake for 30 - 45 minutes. Stir mixture, turning every 15 minutes or until the granola is lightly toasted.
4. Let cool completely before adding the dried fruit and optional ground flaxseeds. Blend to combine.
5. This granola will keep in an airtight container in a cool, dry place for at least 2 weeks.

Makes 1 quart

CHIA SEED PUDDING WITH FRUIT

Chia seeds are a superfood: they are rich in antioxidants, fiber, and iron, which are vital nutrients for cell protection and the elimination of toxins. They are small and compact, yet they have an awesome nutritional profile! Enjoy this highly nutritious dish for breakfast, lunch, or as a dessert with low-sugar fruits like blackberries, blueberries, or raspberries.

The fruit can be added as you are making it or after the pudding has thickened. For maximum flavor, I mixed in the berries right from the start. The following day, I topped the pudding with more fruit. Delicious, and it takes only minutes to make!

INGREDIENTS:

1 cup blackberries
3 tablespoons chia seeds
1 cup almond milk or any non-dairy milk
½ teaspoon cinnamon
½ teaspoon vanilla extract

PREPARATION:

1. Place the berries in a bowl, mash them well and set aside.
2. In a small bowl, combine the chia seeds, milk, cinnamon, and vanilla extract. Add the mashed berries to mixture, mixing well to ensure no clumps.
3. Cover and refrigerate for at least 30 minutes (or overnight) for the best result. After refrigerating, scoop into a jar, bowl, or glass and top with fruit, granola, or other toppings.

Makes 12 ounces

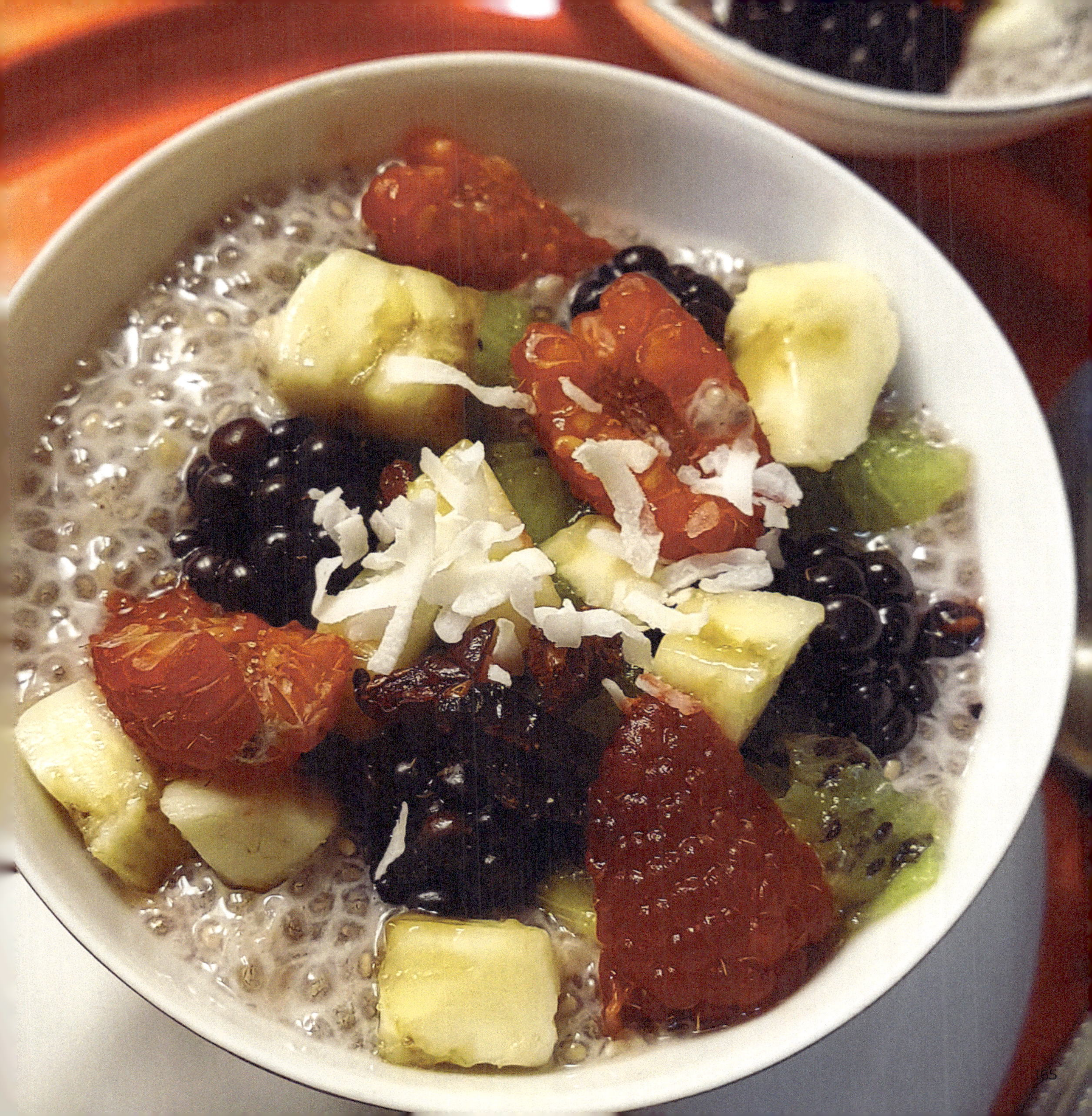

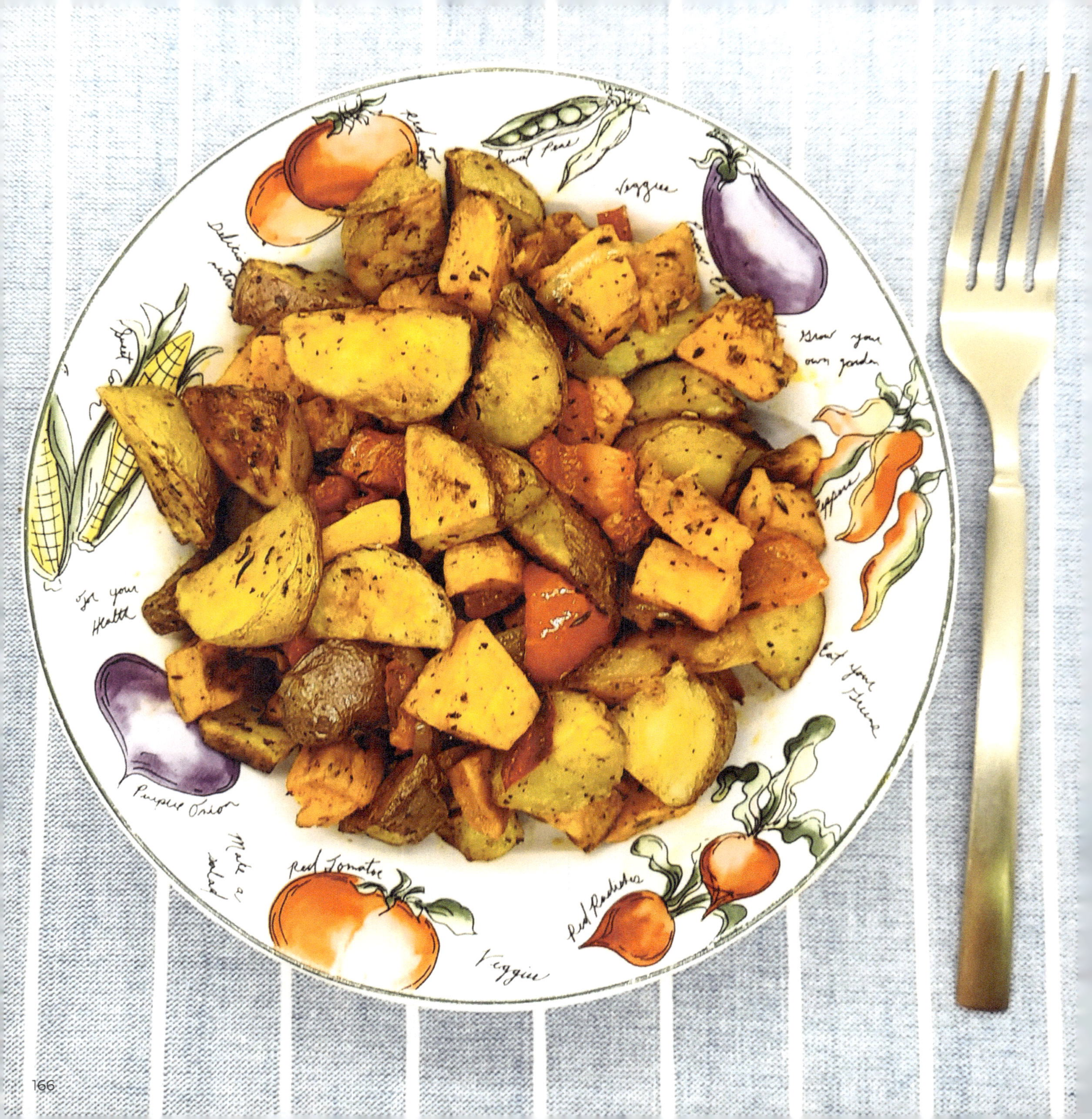
Veggies
Grow your
own garden
Peppers
For your
Health
Purple Onion
Make a
salad
Red Tomatoes
Red Radishes
Veggie

OVEN-ROASTED POTATO - VEGGIE SKILLET

Select your potatoes and veggies, then add herbs and spices for even more flavor! This skillet of oven-roasted potatoes is an excellent source of potassium and can cook itself if you just keep a watchful eye on it. The result is a morning comfort food, especially when you top it with salsa.

INGREDIENTS:
2-3 each Yukon gold, red potatoes cut into equal-size chunks
1 sweet potato, cut in equal-size chunks
1 teaspoon olive oil
½ teaspoon smoked paprika
2 teaspoon dried herb (basil or thyme)
1 bell pepper, chopped
1 onion, quartered
Celtic sea salt and pepper to taste
Optional: Sauce or Salsa (Page 203) for topping

PREPARATION: Pre-heat oven to 425°F.

1. Place potatoes in a bowl and add the oil, smoked paprika, and dried herb. Toss well to coat.

2. Arrange the potatoes in an oven-proof pan or cast-iron skillet and roast for 15 minutes.

3. Turn the potatoes over, add the bell pepper and onion, return to oven to roast 15 more minutes . Check them occasionally to assure all are cooking well and none of them are burning. Potatoes are done when tender to the touch of a fork.

4. If you like, serve with Sauce or salsa.

Makes 4 servings

CHICKPEA SCRAMBLE WITH VEGGIES

I serve this dish for breakfast or brunch along with seasonal fruits and leafy greens. The peppers add a healthy brightness and the mushrooms are a transformative element in this dish, adding a chewy texture and protein. (Mushrooms also contain selenium, phosphorus, calcium, iron, and vitamin B complex.) Chickpeas (a.k.a. garbanzo beans) are very high in protein and fiber. Spinach is super nutritious and gives a comfort that brings you back for more!

INGREDIENTS:

1 teaspoon coconut oil
½ of a small onion, diced (1/4 cup)
5 button mushrooms, sliced
½ of a red bell pepper, diced
2 cups cooked garbanzo beans or one 15-ounce can of garbanzo beans
½ teaspoon ground turmeric
¼ teaspoon ground ginger
¼ teaspoon smoked paprika
1 teaspoon nutritional yeast
Dash of black pepper and Celtic sea salt
Optional: Handful of fresh curly spinach

PREPARATION:

1. In a medium skillet over low heat, warm the coconut oil. Add the onion, mushrooms, and bell pepper. Sauté for 3 minutes, then cover and turn off the heat.

2. For can chickpeas, drain, rinse and mash chickpeas with a fork or use a small chopper.

3. Place the mashed chickpeas in a bowl and stir in the spices, nutritional yeast, pepper, and salt. Mix well. Add water 1 tablespoon at a time until you reach your desired consistency.

4. Turn the heat back on, to a low setting. Blend the chickpea mixture with the vegetables in the skillet, stir well to combine. If using fresh spinach, stir it in now and cook for 1 minute, then cut off heat as the spinach wilts. Serve immediately.

Makes 2 servings

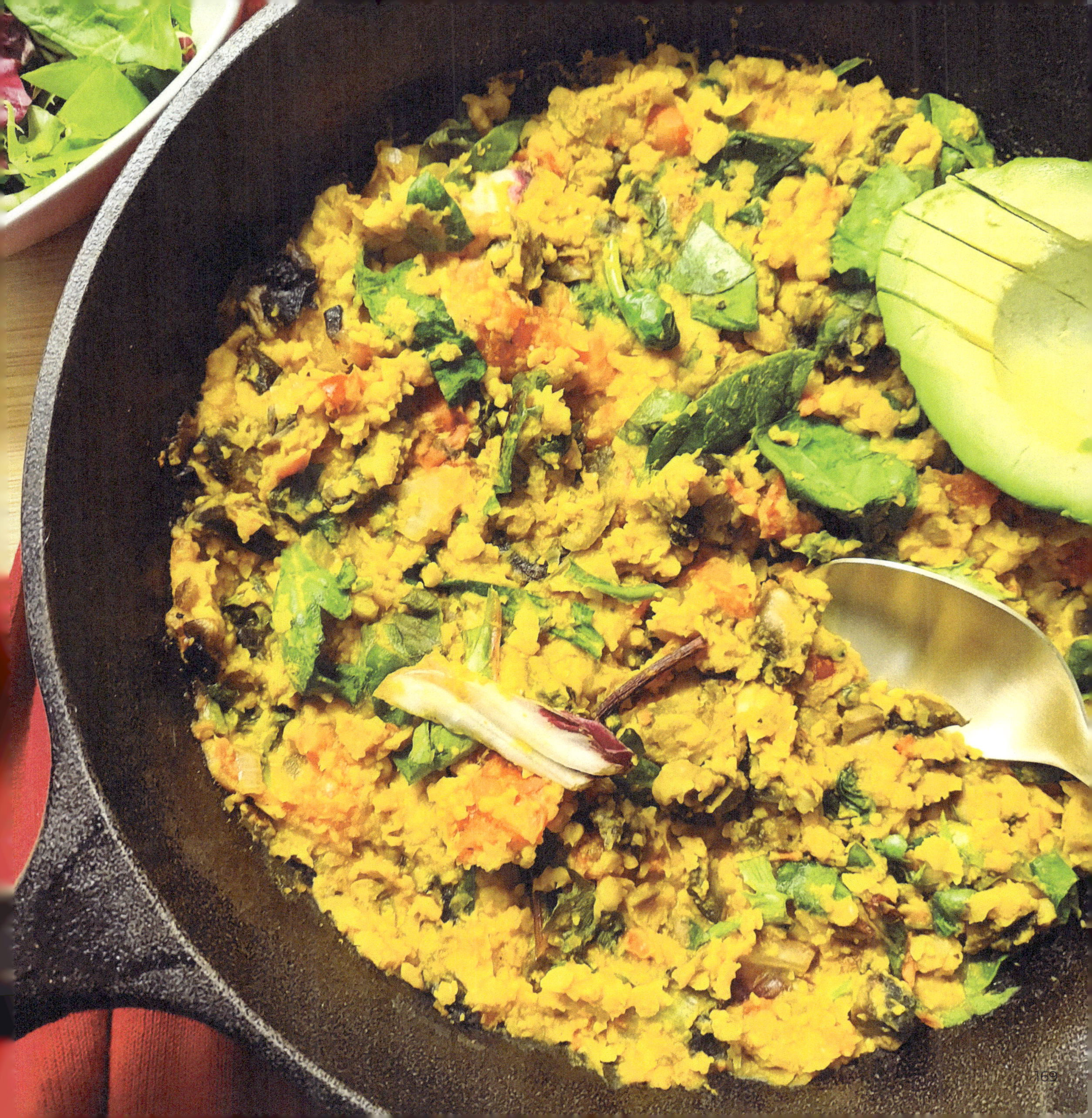

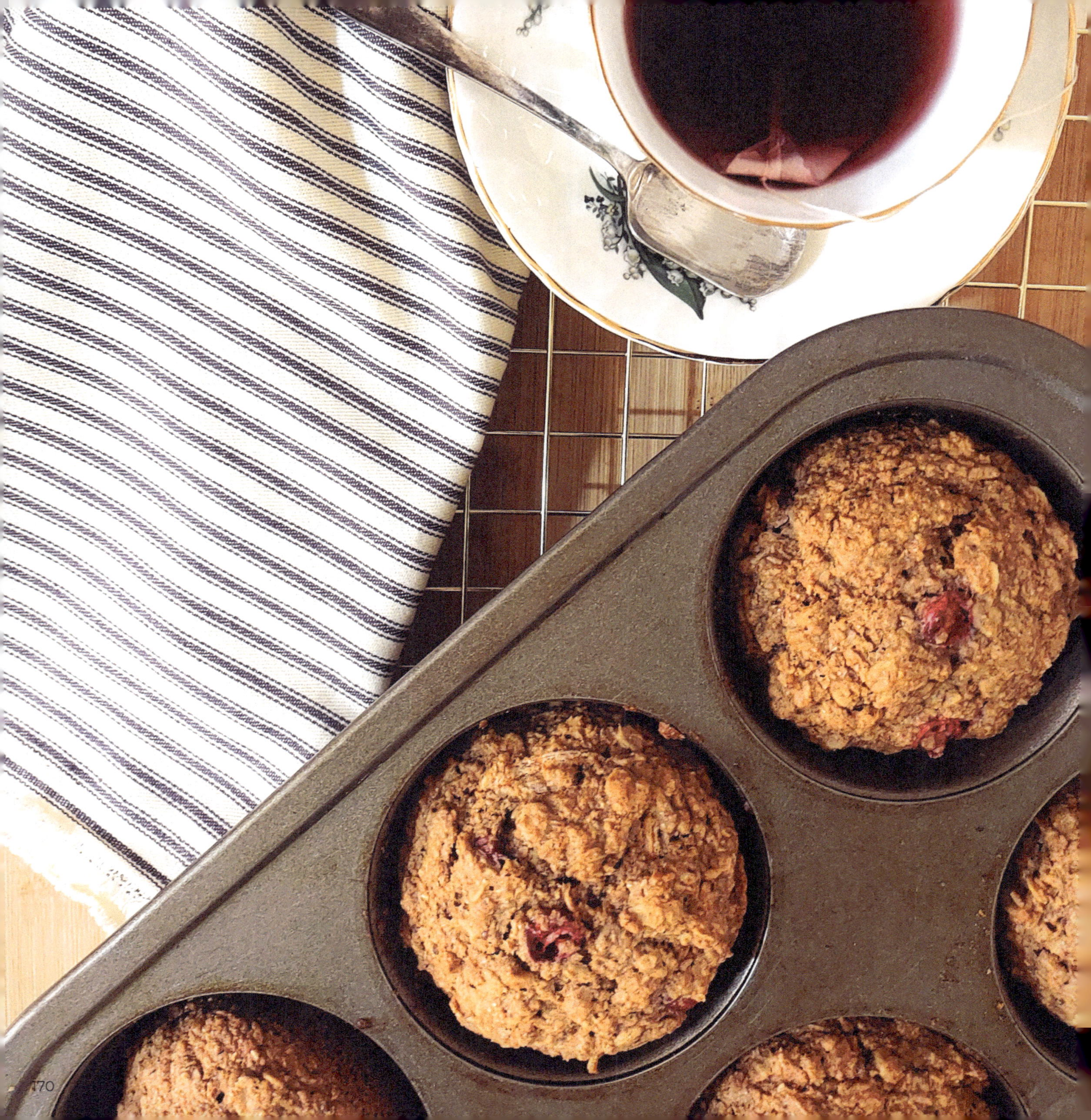

BREAKFAST MUFFINS

Spelt flour is popular because it is very tasty and easy to work with. In these muffins, you get the flavor and nutritional benefits of the whole-grain flour (plus the flaxseed) without dramatically compromising the final texture of the muffins. Spelt is somewhat higher in protein than wheat flour is, although like wheat flour, it contains gluten. Apples give the muffins a moistness. My family loves these muffins and so will you!

INGREDIENTS:

1 tablespoon ground flaxseeds
1½ cups spelt flour
½ cup rolled oats
2 teaspoons aluminum-free baking powder
1 teaspoon baking soda
1 teaspoon ground ginger
1 teaspoon ground allspice
1 teaspoon ground cinnamon
¼ teaspoon ground nutmeg
½ teaspoon Celtic Sea salt
½ cup almond milk
(or any non-dairy milk)
1 teaspoon vanilla extract
¼ cup honey
1/3 cup olive oil
1 small apple, grated
1 small carrot, grated
Fresh Cranberries, Optional
Variation: ½ cup blueberries can
be substitute

PREPARATION: Preheat oven to 400°F.

1. In a small bowl, mix the ground flaxseeds with 3 tablespoons of water. Let stand for 3 minutes to thicken.
2. In large mixing bowl, add the flour, oats, baking powder, baking soda, spices, and salt. In a medium bowl, whisk together the milk, vanilla, honey, oil, and flaxseed mixture.
3. Combine the wet ingredients and dry ingredients. Add grated apple and carrot and mix into the batter until just combined.
4. Fill each muffin tin ¾ full with batter. Bake 20 minutes or until an inserted toothpick comes out clean. Allow to cool.

Makes 6 large or 12 regular muffins

APRICOT - APPLE SPREAD

This summery, sunny orange apricot spread is full of beta-carotene! It is a delightful and delicious spread, wonderful on muffins or toast or when served as a condiment with summer meals.

INGREDIENTS:
3 apples, peels and cores removed, chopped
3 pitted apricots, chopped
1 cinnamon stick
½ teaspoon ground ginger
¼ teaspoon vanilla extract
Optional: Maple syrup

PREPARATION:

1. Place all ingredients except the maple syrup in a medium-size pot and add 2 tablespoons of water.
2. Bring to a boil, then reduce heat to low and simmer for 15 minutes or until the fruit is soft. Add more water if the mixture starts to stick to the pot.
3. Remove the cooked mixture and mash well. Sweeten if you like.

Makes 1 cup

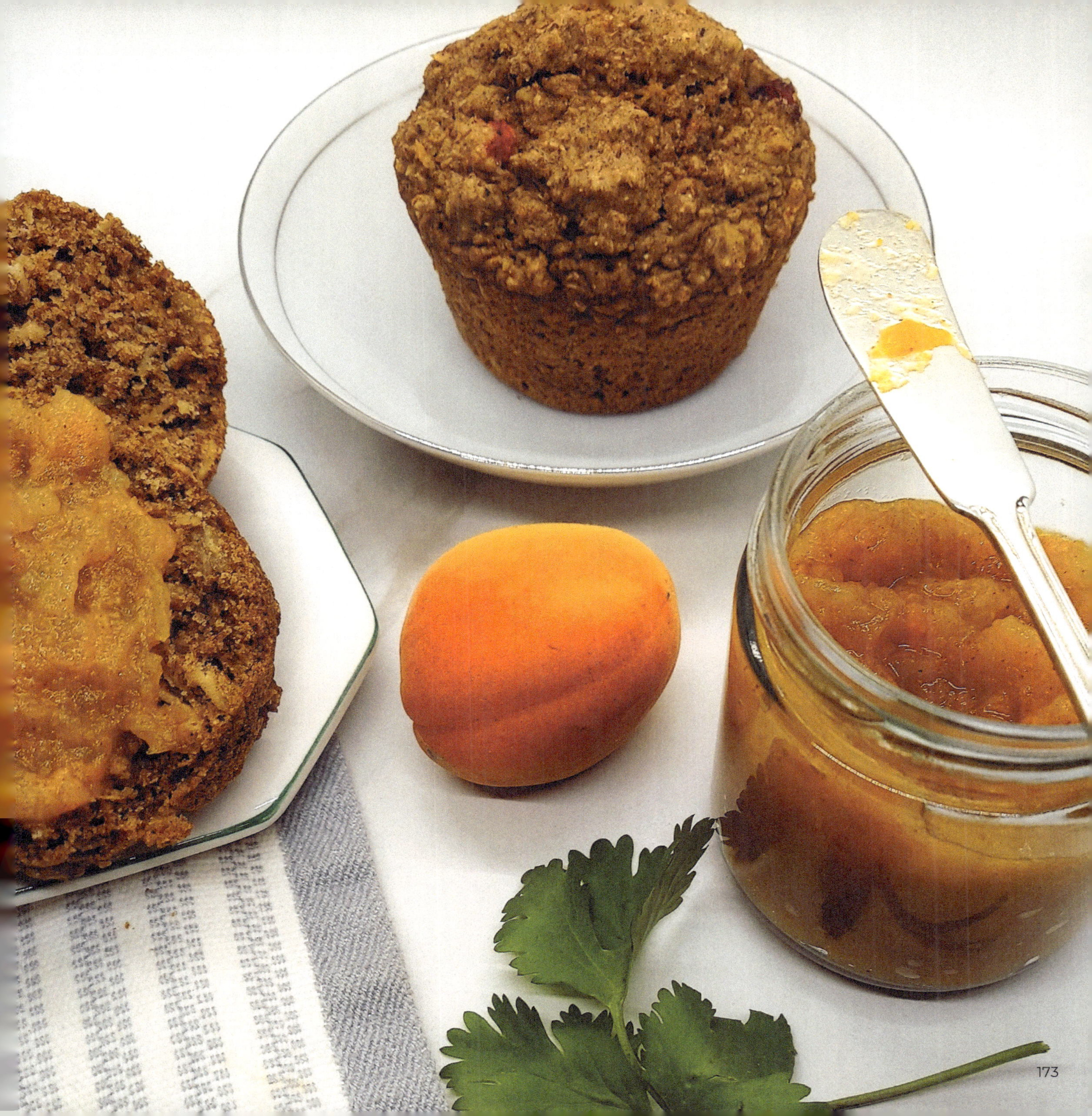

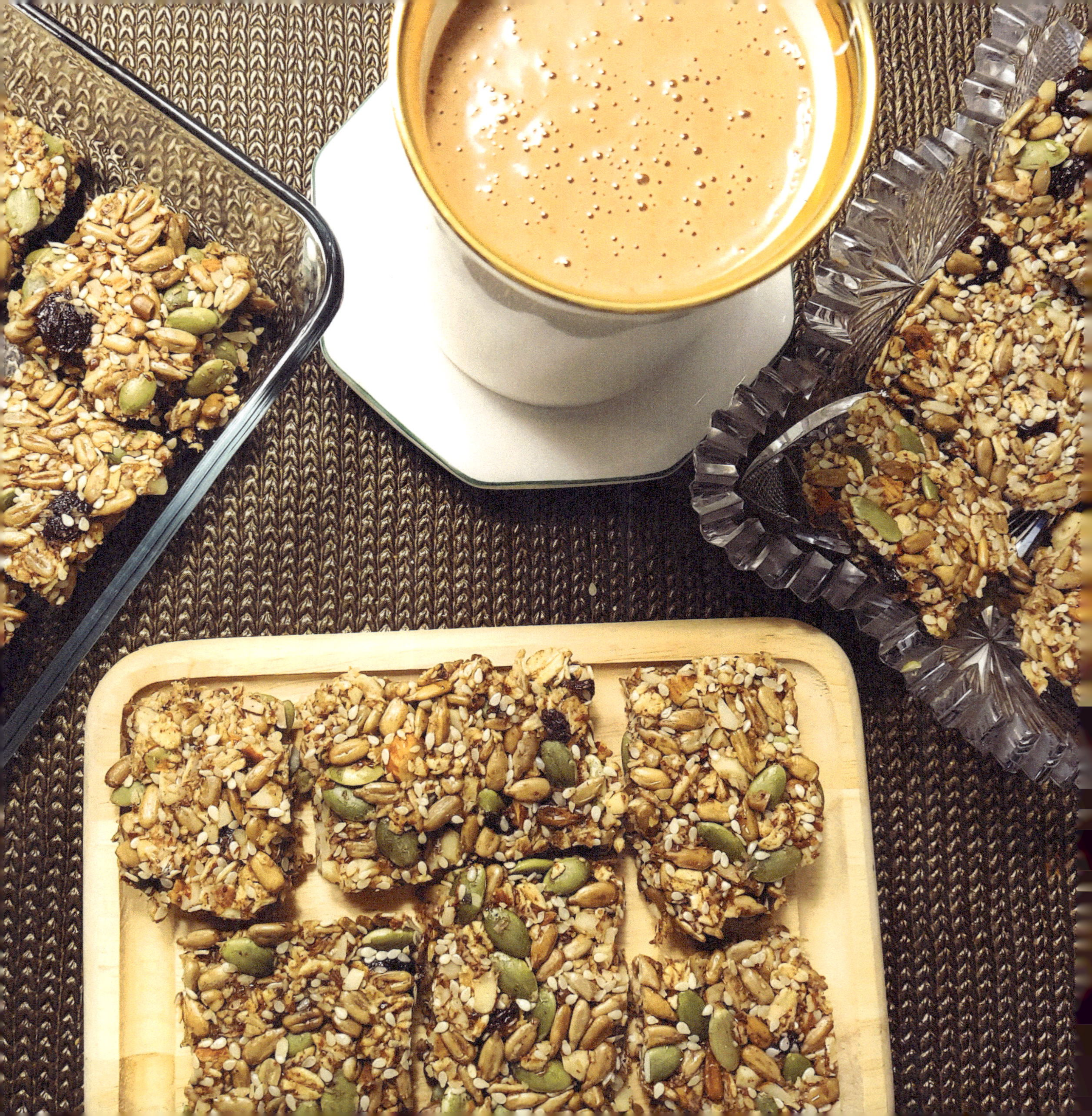

NUT AND SEED ENERGY CHEWS

Seeds and nuts are some of the most concentrated forms of vitamins, minerals, nutrients, and essential fatty acids we can get in our diet. Although each type of seed and nut is unique, many share the same amino acids and omega-3 fatty acids, and all contain fiber as well. When you add in their vitamin and protein content, you have a complete dietary staple that can have a wide range of positive effects on the body.

INGREDIENTS:
2 tablespoons ground flaxseeds
¼ cup raw almonds, coarsely chopped
½ cup raw pumpkin seeds
1 cup raw sunflower seeds
¼ cup sesame seeds
½ cup rolled oats
1 teaspoon ground cinnamon
1/3 cup raisins
1 large overripe banana, mashed

1½ tablespoons maple syrup
1 tablespoon coconut oil, melted
1 teaspoon vanilla extract

PREPARATION: Pre-heat oven to 325°F.

1. In a small bowl, mix ground flaxseeds with 5 tablespoons of water. Let stand for 3 minutes to thicken.
2. Place the nuts, seeds, oats, spice and raisins in a large bowl. Add to the mashed banana- the syrup, oil, vanilla and the flaxseed mixture. And blend well,
3. Line a rimmed baking sheet with parchment paper. Pour the mixture onto the parchment paper and smooth with wooden spoon. Lay a second parchment sheet over the mixture covering completely, then press the mixture evenly spreading it into the corners and sides of the pan.
4. Place the baking sheet in oven and bake for 20-30 minutes. The chews are done when they turn golden brown around the edges. Remove from oven and allow to cool. When cool to the touch, cut into pieces.

Makes 3 dozen bite-sized chews

RED RUSSIAN KALE SMOOTHIE

Red Russian kale is a beautiful purple color and is a rich source of vitamin C, beta-carotene, calcium, lutein, zeaxanthin, magnesium, potassium, protein, and fiber. For this smoothie, I add flax or chia seeds for the anti-inflammatory omega-3 fatty acid and avocado for the healthy fat. Fat is necessary for our bodies to transform beta-carotene into vitamin A.

INGREDIENTS:
3-4 leaves red Russian kale
1 banana, frozen or fresh
½ of an avocado
1 tablespoon ground flaxseeds or whole chia seeds
½ teaspoon ground cinnamon
2 cups almond milk

PREPARATION:

Place kale, bananas, avocado, flax seeds,cinnamon and milk in a high-speed blender or nutri-bullet and blend until totally smooth.

Makes 24 ounces

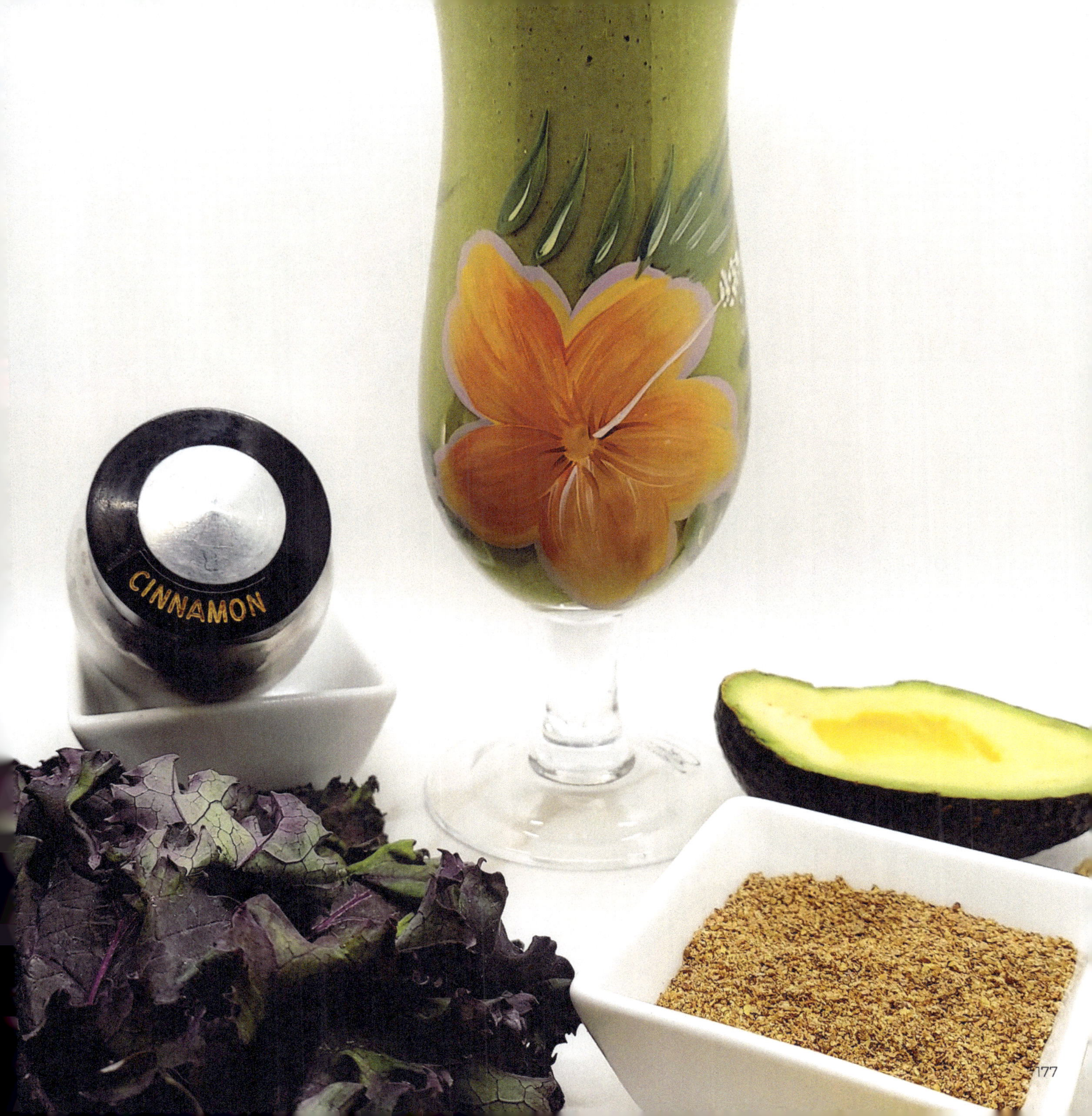
CINNAMON

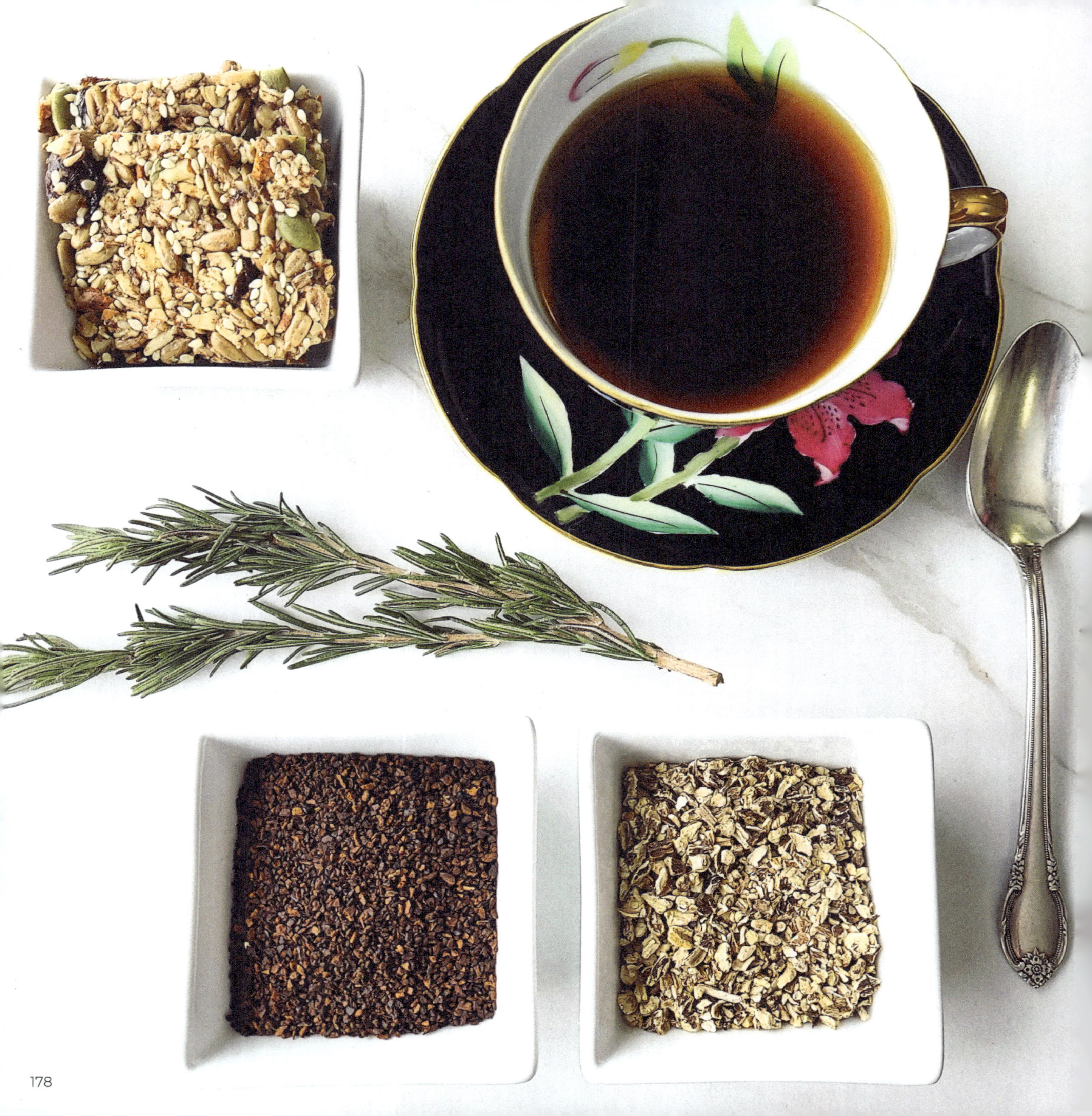

ROAST CHICORY & DANDELION ROOT DRINK

If you crave a wonderful caffeine-free coffee alternative, chicory root and dandelion root will do the job!! Like coffee, these roots have a robust flavor and aroma. Chicory is a member of the dandelion family and has a high fiber content along with other nutrients. Dandelion root is a good source of beta-carotene, and the flowering plant is rich in vitamin C, fiber, potassium, iron, calcium. magnesium, zinc, and phosphorus.

INGREDIENTS:

3 cardamom pods (or ½ teaspoon ground cardamon)
1 teaspoon roasted chicory root granules
2 tablespoons roasted dandelion root
Optional: Your choice of sweetener

PREPARATION:

1. Crush the cardamom pods and place in a cup. Add the chicory root and dandelion root. Pour 2 cups of boiling water over them and let steep for 4 minutes.
2. Pour through a strainer into another cup. Discard the solids and serve immediately as is or with sweetener of your choice.

Makes 2 cups (12 ounces)

CACAO HOT CHOCOLATE

This super-chocolatey delight is made with organic raw (sugar-free) cacao powder. Raw cacao is said to be the richest source of magnesium on the planet. Chocolate comes from the cacao bean. Add raw cacao powder to smoothies and used in other dishes and desserts as in the Cacao Avocado Pie (page 227).

INGREDIENTS:

1½ cups non-dairy milk of your choice
1 -1/2 tablespoons raw organic cacao powder
½ teaspoon vanilla extract
½ teaspoon ground cinnamon
Drizzle of maple syrup

PREPARATION:

1. Place all ingredients in a small pot and heat gently, stirring well to combine. Pour into cups and enjoy.
2. The Coconut Cream Topping (page 228)

Makes 2 servings

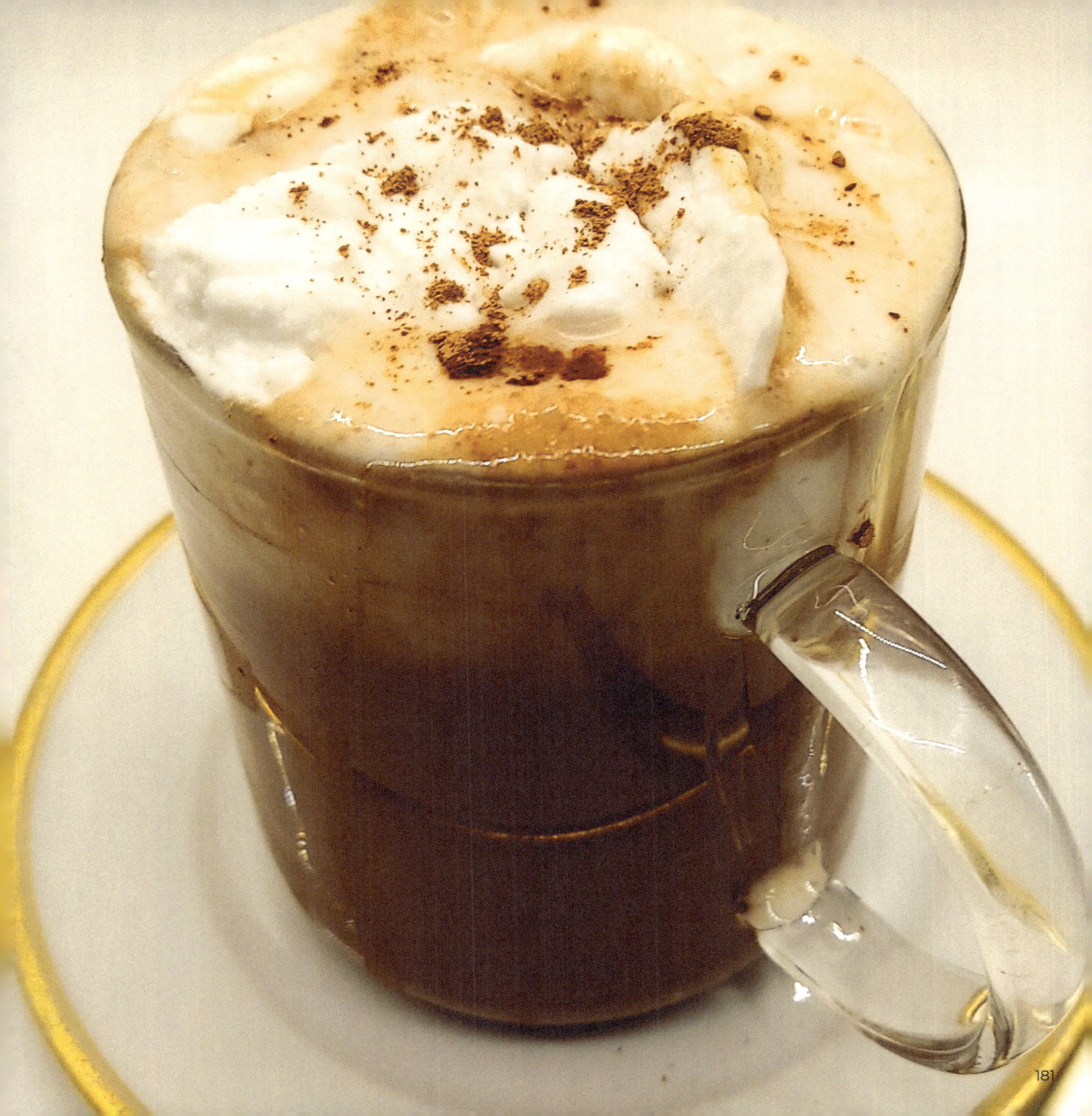

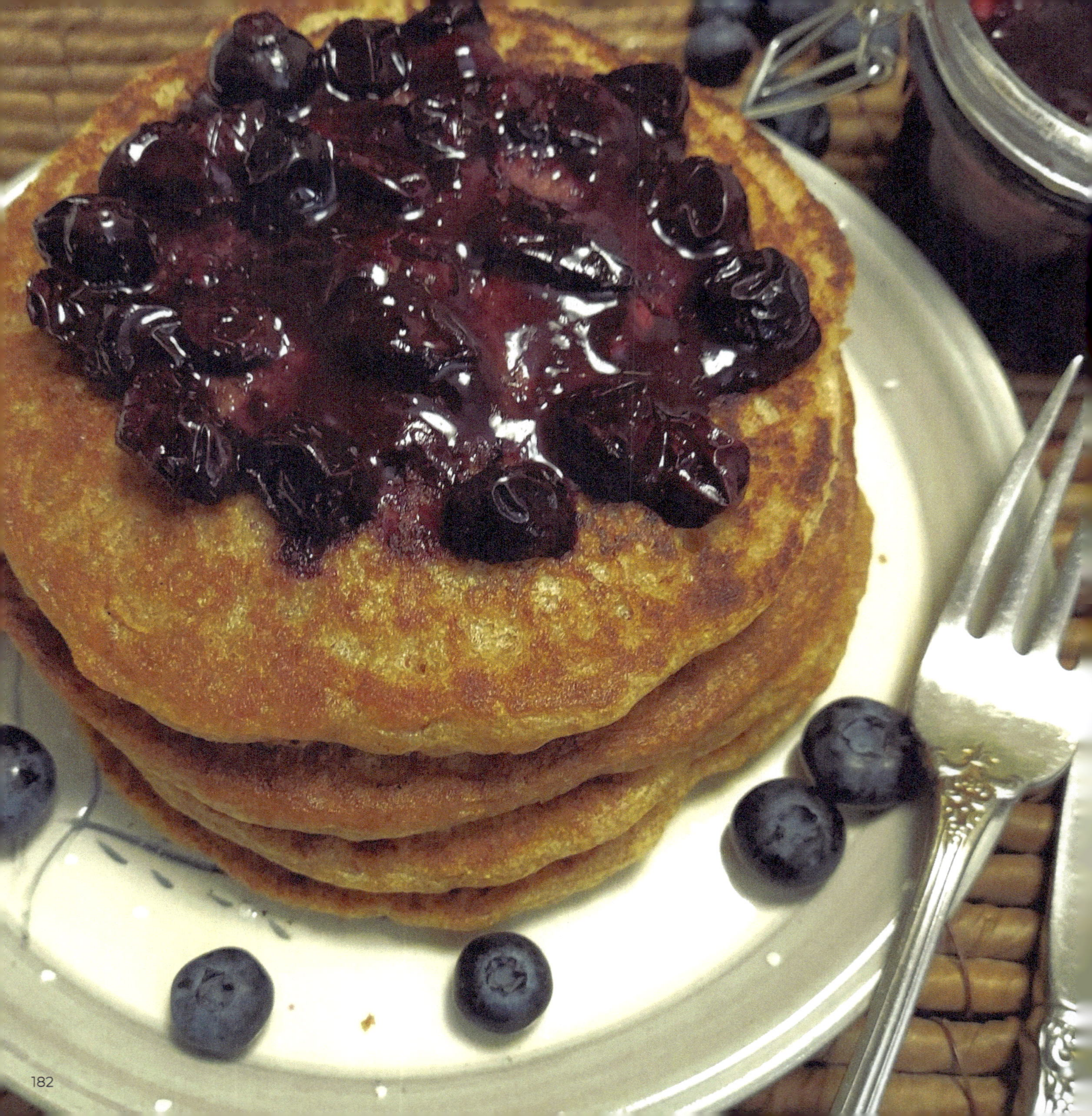

VEGAN BUTTERMILK PANCAKES

While working on this recipe – I had an aha moment - remembering buttermilk was/is known as a secret ingredient in baking. Light, fluffy pancakes are a great breakfast option.

INGREDIENTS:
1 cup almond milk (or any non-dairy milk)
1 lemon, juiced (approx.3 tablespoons)
1 cup spelt flour (or buckwheat flour)
2 teaspoon aluminum free baking powder
½ teaspoon baking soda
1 tablespoon coconut sugar
1/4 teaspoon celtic sea salt
2 teaspoon coconut oil (for the pan)
Optional: Blueberry compote (page 184)

PREPARATION:

1. In a small bowl add the milk and lemon juice, mix and allow to stand for ten minutes. The result is a vegan version of buttermilk. Tip: the ten minutes are necessary
2. In a medium size bowl, mix the flour, baking powder, baking soda, sugar and salt together. Pour the wet ingredients into the dry ingredients, mix lightly and evenly. Allow batter to sit 5 minutes.
3. Warm the coconut oil in a skillet (cast iron) or grill and scoop pancake batter onto the pan. Cook couple minutes as bubbles form around the edges, then flip, cook on other side until done.
4. Enjoy with your favorite syrup, preserves or the optional blueberry compote

Makes 4-6 pancakes

BLUEBERRY COMPOTE

I love pancakes moistened with the sweetness of fruit! Blueberries can easily be reduced to a compote (stewed fruit), leaving the berries intact and you in control of the sweetness. This fancy sounding, quick recipe will add a sparkle to many dishes. Enjoy alone or over waffles, cakes, or as a topping on desserts.

INGREDIENTS:
1 pint fresh blueberries, rinsed
1 teaspoon of fresh lemon juice
½ cup water
Sweetener of your choice, to your taste

PREPARATION:

1. Add the blueberries, water and lemon juice to a small saucepan over low heat. Cook for 5 minutes, notice the berries softening. Stir gently to keep fruit intact.

2. Continue cooking 5 minutes or more as the mixture thickens. It will also thicken as it cools. Store in a covered jar in the refrigerator up to 5 days. Tip: You can also mix an equal amount of arrowroot and water until smooth, then stir into mixture as a thickener.

Makes 2 cups

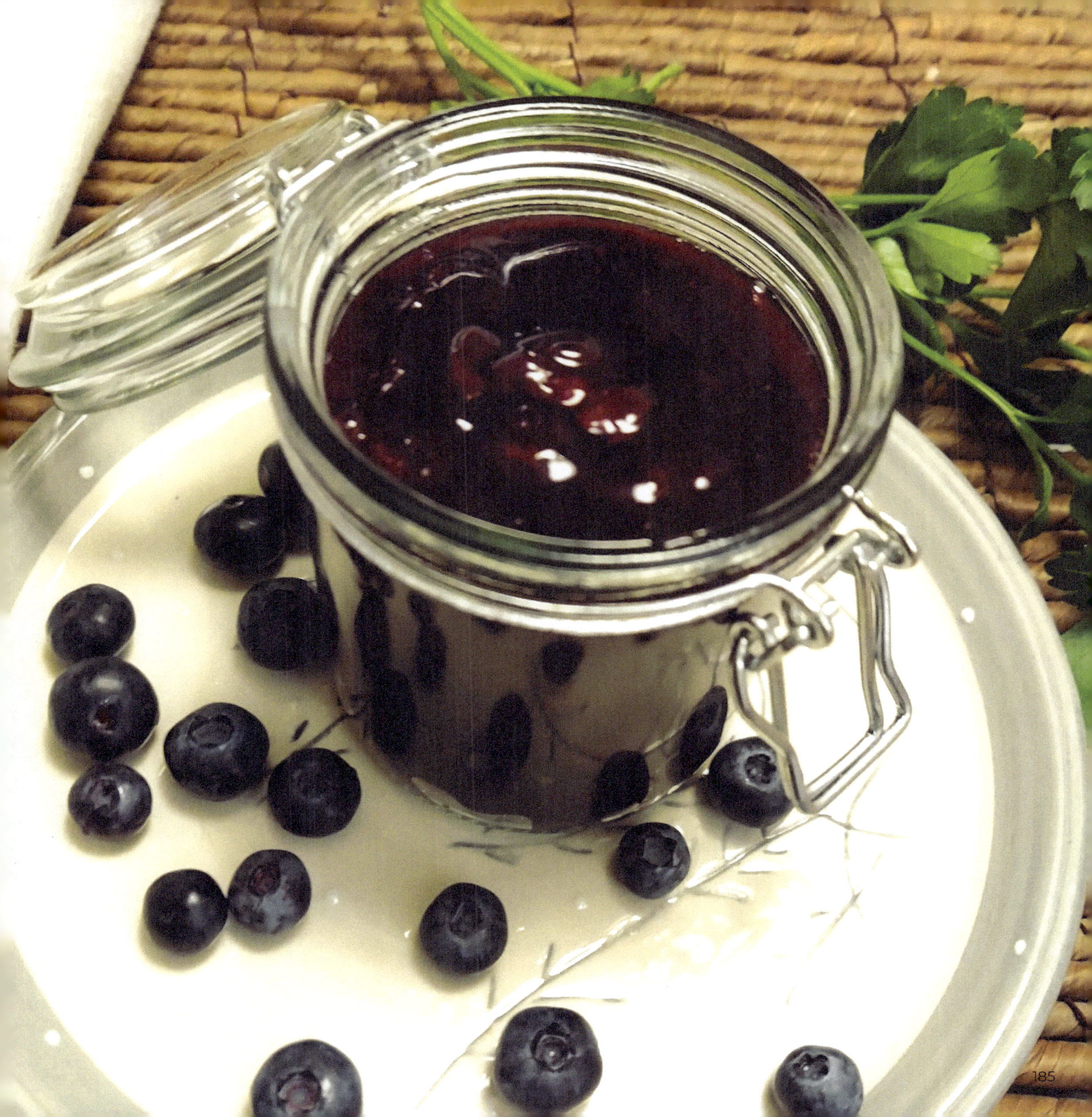

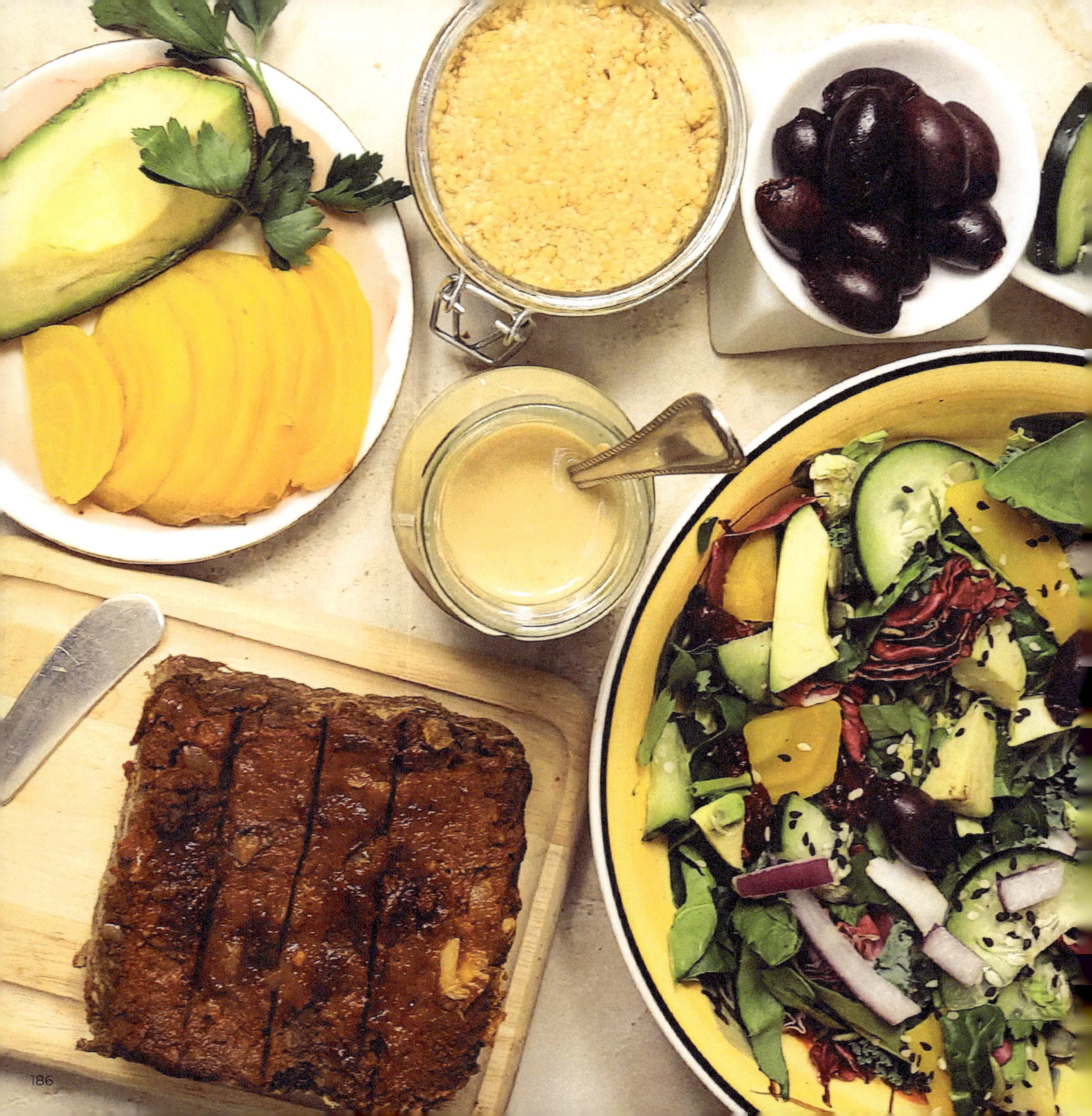

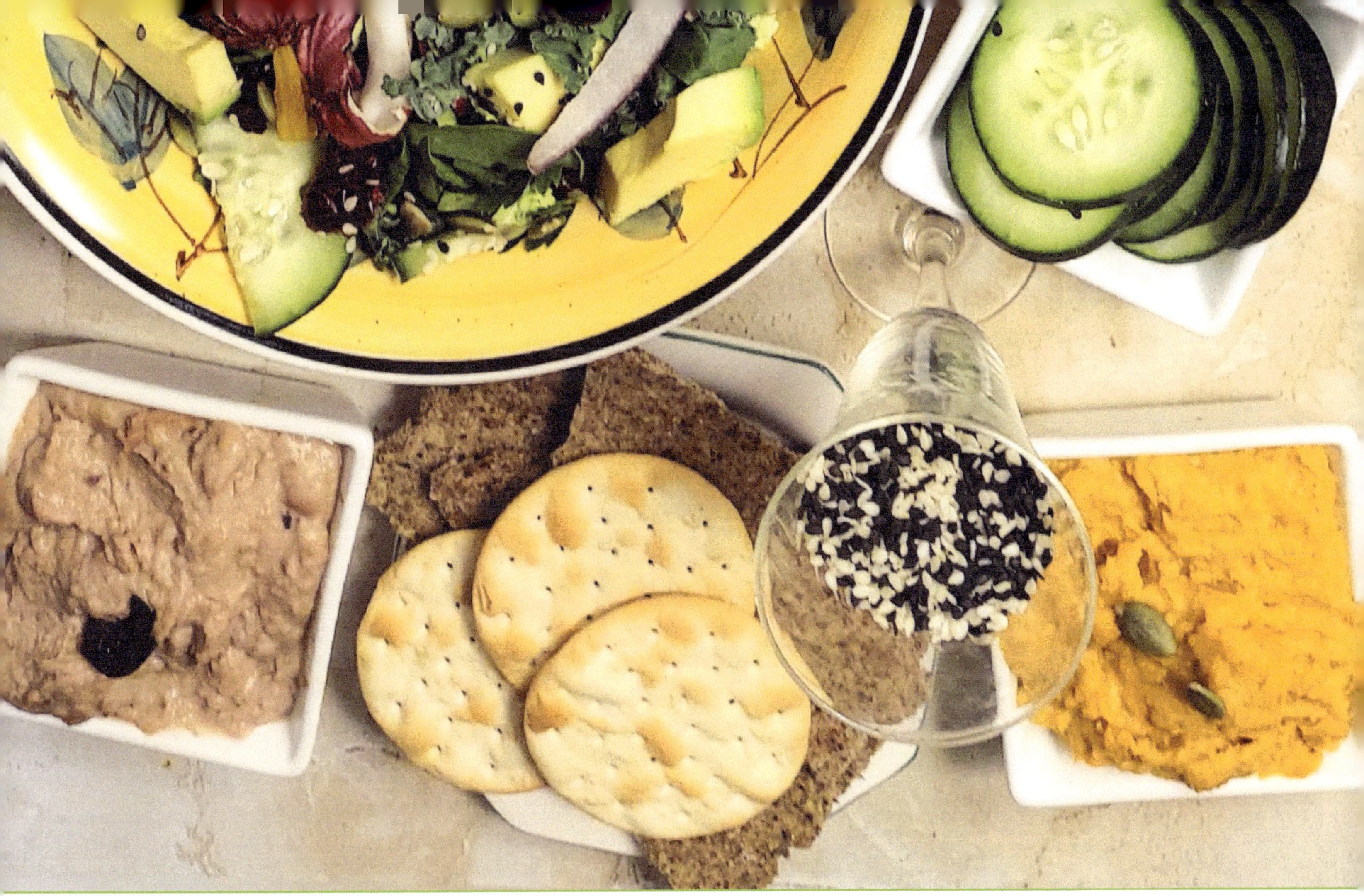

CONDIMENTS AND MORE

CONDIMENTS AND MORE RECIPES

Today, condiments cover a wide selection of food items. This food category is much different from the condiment lists of years ago, which included mustard, ketchup, relish and little more. Tasty ingredients, like sauces, dips, seasonings, dressings, pastes, and more are today popular supplements to a dish or a meal. The plant-based lifestyle, an on-the go lifestyle, is best when introducing variety and flavor that is compact and portable while large on nutritional impact. These foods can also introduce nutrient-rich options to avoid nutrient deficiencies. The options can be as simple as blending a paste, or fermenting a vegetable.

Growing up, my Aunt Betty made Cha-Cha (aka Chow Chow) from her garden vegetables. Cha-Cha, a relish traditionally made of green tomatoes, cabbage, onions, and peppers is a condiment. It was jarred up and served with greens, meats, peas, and beans. The flavors enhanced the dishes it was served with while adding fresh garden vegetables and healthy nutrients.

Salsa is a popular sauce. Traditional salsa blends fresh vegetables with lime juice, red onions, and the herb cilantro. Cilantro leaves are associated with the removal of heavy metals (like mercury, lead, and aluminum) from the body. As I squeeze fresh lime juice, a major source of vitamin C, into a dish of salsa, ultimately, I transfer vitamin C into my body. Vitamin C is said to enhance the absorption of iron in the body. Reflectively, selecting healthy condiments is a great way to boost flavor and add additional nutrition to the diet.

Let's Welcome Condiments and more.

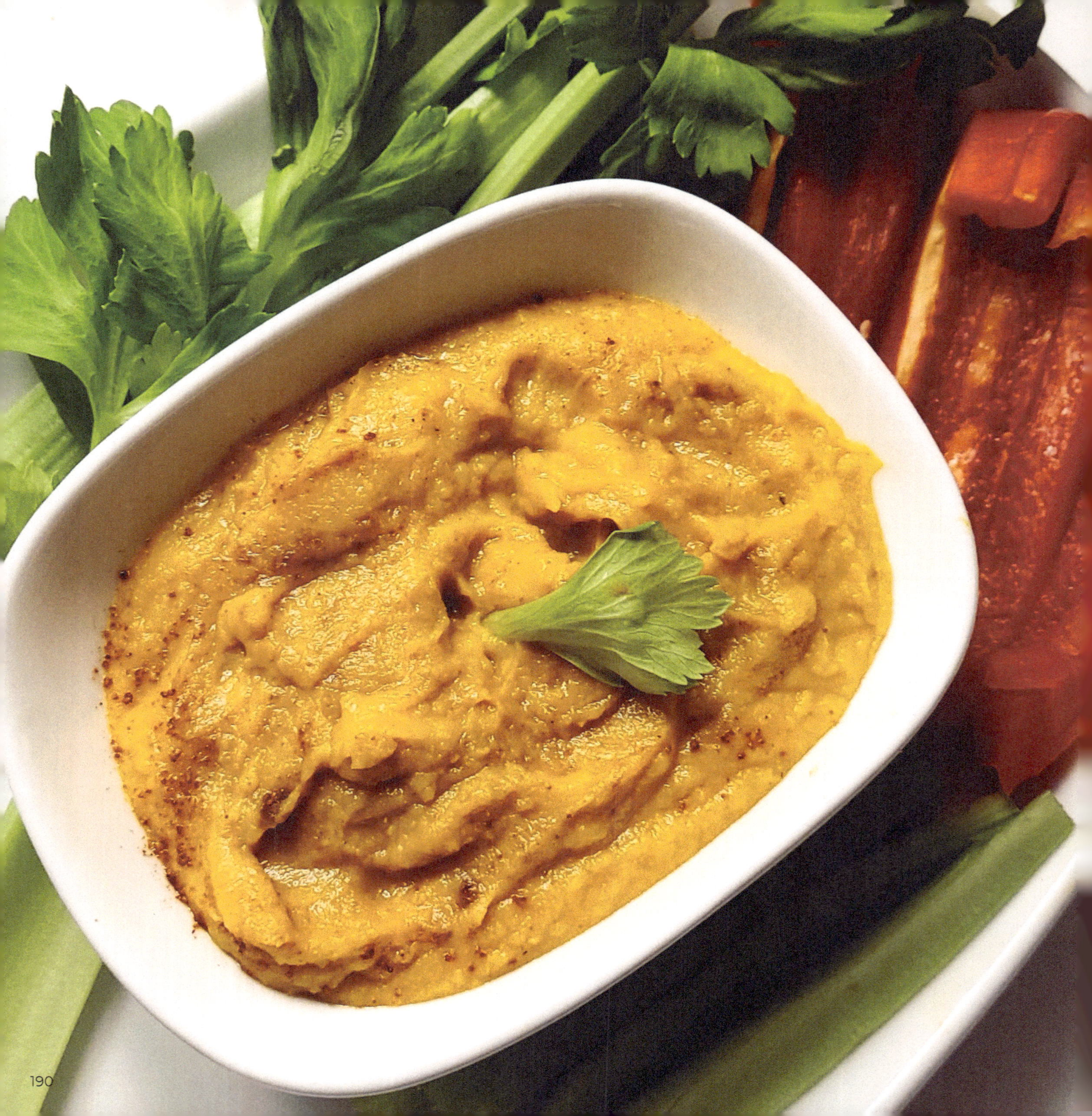

ROASTED SWEET POTATO HUMMUS

The sweetness of the potatoes gives this hummus an untraditional but awesome flavor. Sweet potatoes are an excellent source of beta-carotene (for eye health) and vitamin C.

INGREDIENTS:

2 cups cooked chickpeas or one 15-ounce can of chickpeas
1 large sweet potato, oven-roasted (see box)
1 tablespoon tahini paste
Juice and zest of ½ lemon
1 clove garlic, chopped
2 tablespoons olive oil
2 teaspoons ground cumin
½ teaspoon Celtic sea salt
½ teaspoon smoked paprika

PREPARATION: Pre-heat oven to 400°F.

1. Drain and rinse the chickpeas if you're using canned chickpeas. Place chickpeas in a bowl and mash with a fork.

2. Remove the skin of the sweet potato and mash the flesh until it's smooth. Transfer the mashed sweet potato and chickpeas to a food processor. Add ¼ cup water and all of the remaining ingredients except for the smoked paprika.

3. Blend until smooth, adding water as needed to reach your desired consistency.

4. Scoop into a bowl, sprinkle paprika over the top, and serve.

Makes 12 ounces

OVEN-ROASTING SWEET POTATOES

Scrub the potatoes and rub them with oil.

Place the potatoes on a baking tray and poke a couple of holes in each one.

Roast until they're tender when pierced by fork, about 45 minutes.
Allow to cool.

FLAX CRACKERS

These simple crackers are full of healthy omega-3 fats from flax seeds. They are quick to make and fit for snacks or any occasion!

INGREDIENTS:
½ cup spelt flour
¼ cup ground flaxseeds
½ teaspoon aluminum-free baking powder
½ teaspoon dried thyme or rosemary
Pinch of sea salt
½ tablespoon olive oil

PREPARATION: Pre-heat oven to 400°F.

1. In a small bowl, mix together the flour, flaxseeds, baking powder, dried herbs, and pinch of sea salt.

2. Add ¼ cup water and the oil to ingredients in the bowl. Mix with a spoon, then knead it with your hands.

3. Arrange the dough on parchment paper and use a rolling pin to roll the dough out until it's about ¼" thick.

4. Transfer the parchment paper onto a baking sheet and bake for 8-10 minutes in pre-heated oven or until the edges are browning.

Makes 2 dozen crackers

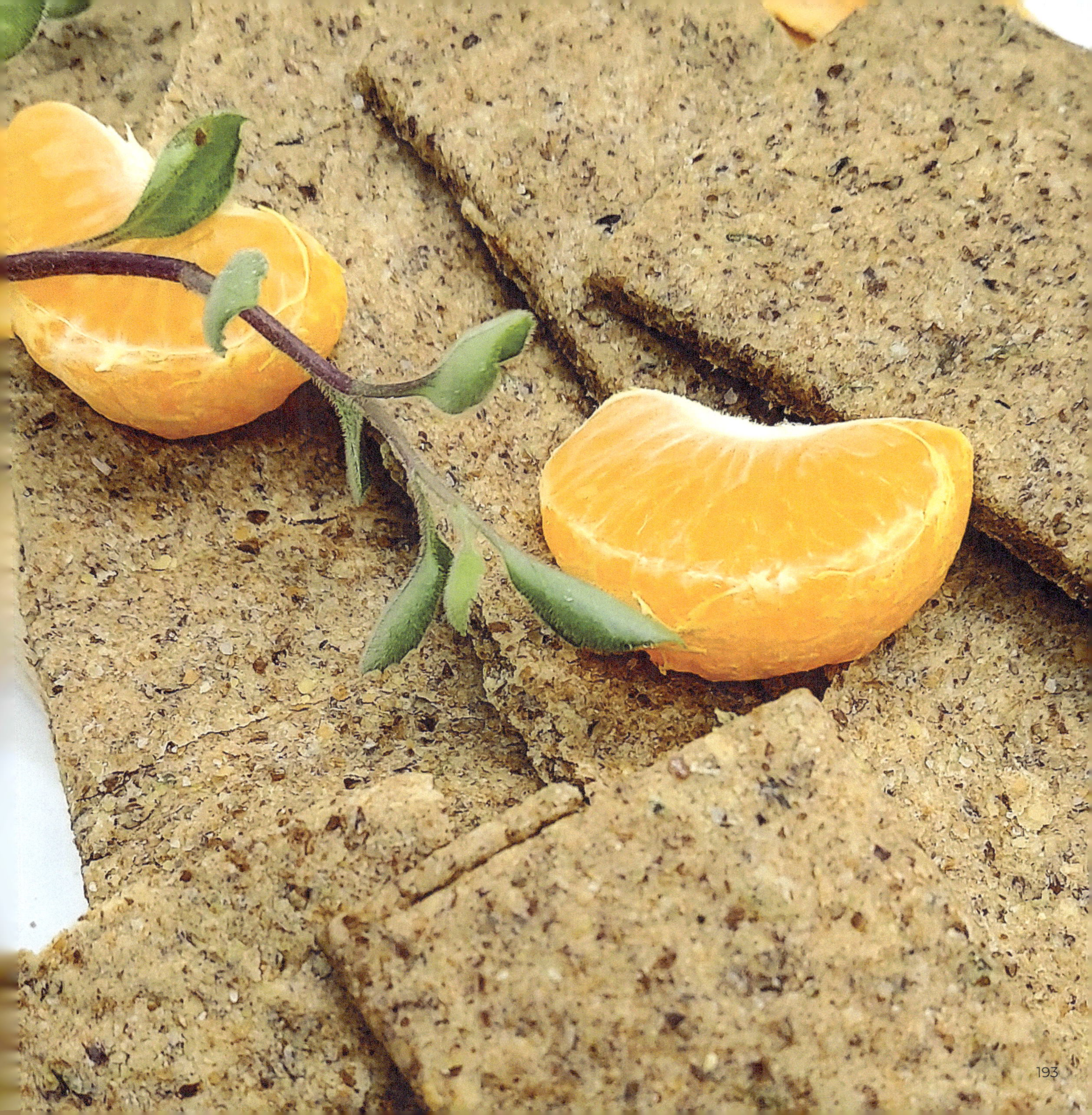

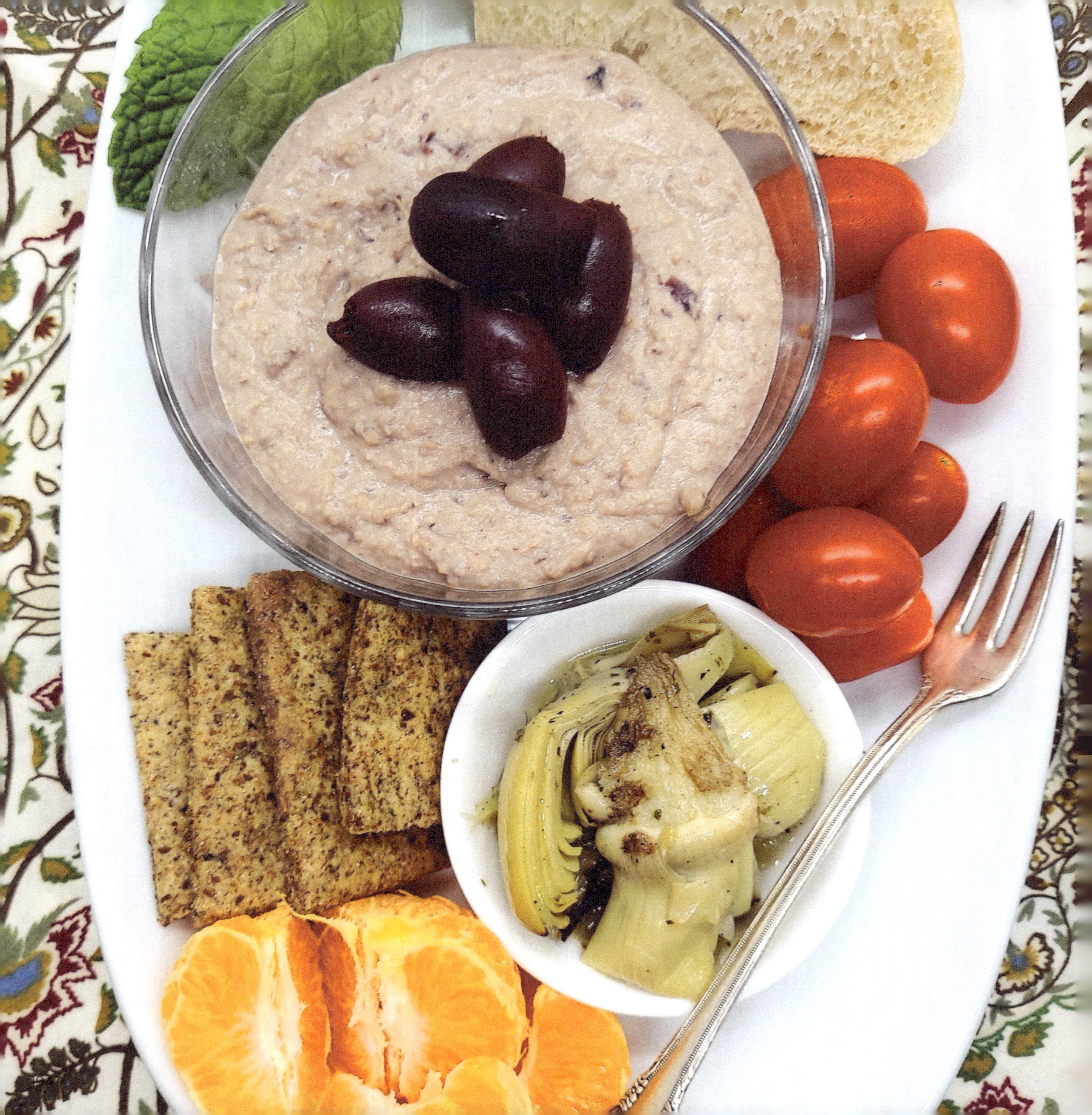

KALAMATA OLIVE HUMMUS

This spread is a favorite of mine. When I could no longer find kalamata olive hummus on grocery shelves, I took to the kitchen. This savory, smoky appetizer can be served with crackers or crudités.

INGREDIENTS:

2 cups cooked chickpeas, or one 15-ounce can of chickpeas
2 tablespoons tahini paste
1 clove garlic, chopped
2 tablespoons fresh lemon juice
8 pitted Kalamata olives
¼ teaspoon of Celtic sea salt

PREPARATION:

Place all ingredients in a high-speed blender and add ¼ cup water. Blend until smooth. Store in airtight container in refrigerator.

Makes 10 ounces

WHOLE-GRAIN MUSTARD

Finding a good mustard to use to flavor a salad dressing or to use as a condiment was a chore. Years ago, I tried making my own...and I've never looked back. Mustard seeds are from the brassica family (which includes broccoli, collards, etc.), meaning that mustard is an anti-inflammatory spice and a flavorful one. Yellow mustard seeds are milder than brown mustard seeds, so for a more spicy flavor, mix 1/3 cup each of yellow and brown mustard seeds (equal parts= 2/3 cup). Tip: The liquid we use must be at a cool temperature for the mustard seeds to become a smooth emulsification.

INGREDIENTS:
2/3 cup yellow mustard seeds
2/3 cup apple cider vinegar
1 tablespoon honey

PREPARATION:

1. In a small bowl, add the mustard seeds and 2/3 cup cold water. Let sit for 10 minutes before adding the vinegar. Cover the bowl and let it stand at room temperature for 12 hours.

2. Transfer the mixture to a blender and add the honey. Blend to your desired consistency (i.e., smooth or coarse).

3. Store mustard in a clean glass container. Chill at least 3 days before serving. Mustard can be stored in the refrigerator up to 5 months in an airtight container.

Makes 12 ounces

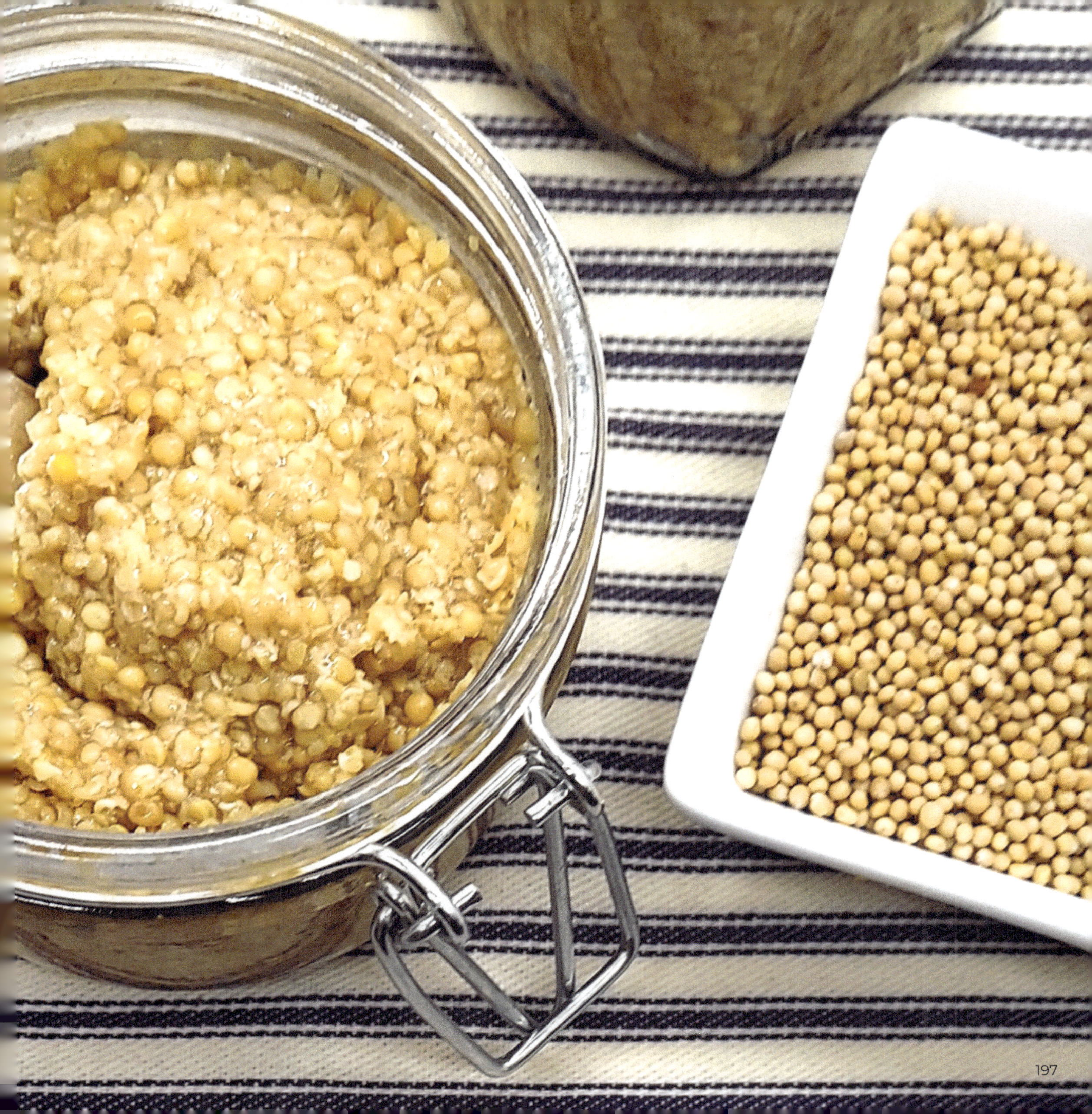

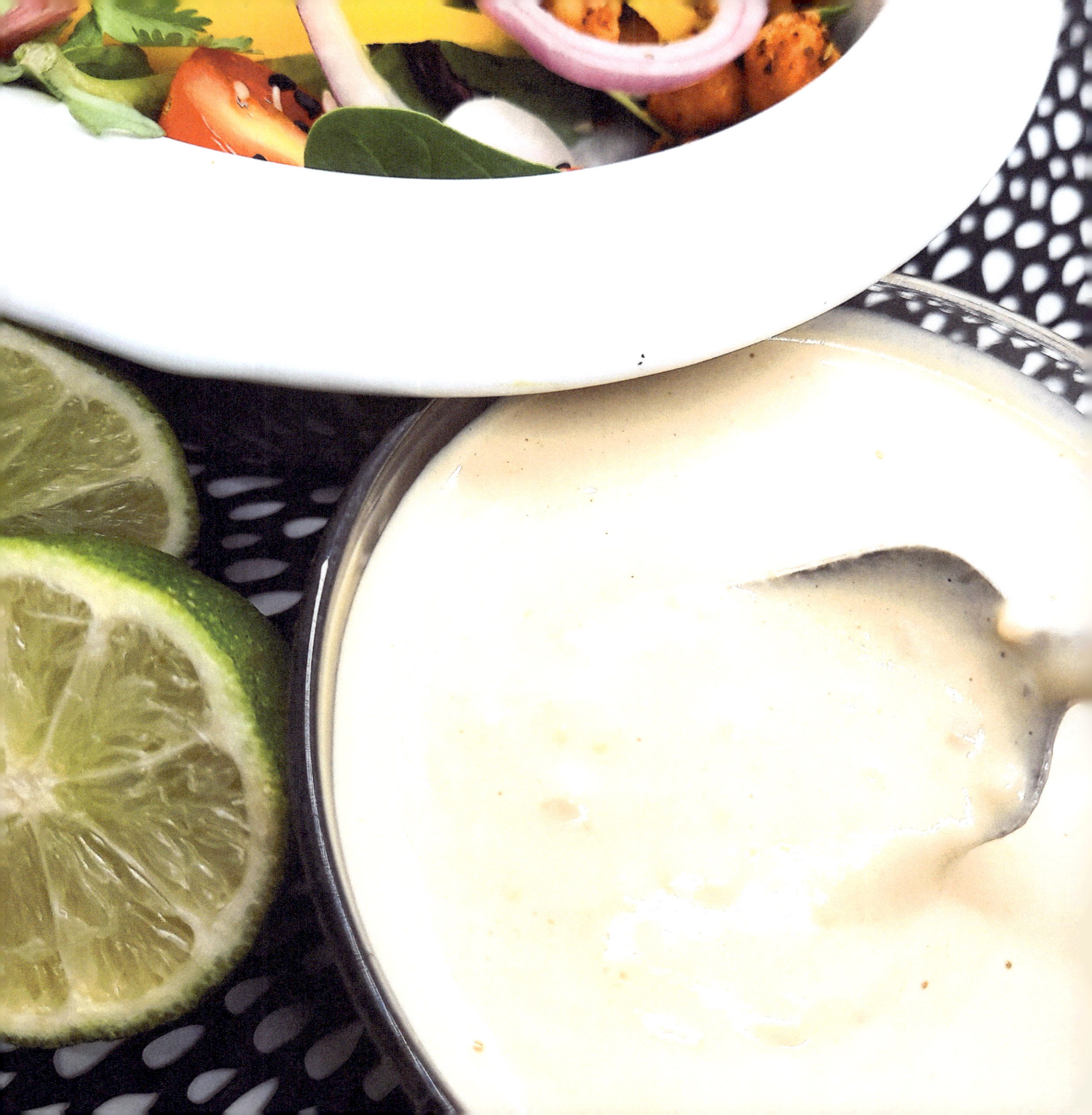

TAHINI-LIME DRESSING

Tahini paste is made of toasted sesame seeds that are ground until they have the consistency of a nut butter. Here again are sesame seeds, tiny and super rich in copper, magnesium, and calcium. Tahini dressing blends well with salads as well as vegetable dishes as a multi-purpose, nutrient rich, gluten-free dressing.

INGREDIENTS:
1/2 cup tahini paste
1 teaspoon ground ginger
¼ cup fresh lime juice
2 teaspoons whole-grain mustard (page xx)
1 tablespoon maple syrup
¼ teaspoon of Celtic Sea salt

PREPARATION:

1. Place the tahini in a small bowl and stir in the ginger, lime juice, mustard, maple syrup, salt and ¼ cup water. Blend until smooth

2. Leftover dressing will last for 5 days in the refrigerator.

Makes 1 cup

BEV'S BBQ SAUCE

This tangy barbecue sauce is very versatile and is the perfect flavor enhancer for many dishes. Plus, it is quick, easy to make, and allows you to control the ingredients. This can be a template to add your favorite spices. I use this sauce in place of ketchup.

INGREDIENTS:

1 teaspoon olive oil
2 tablespoons minced onion
2 cloves garlic
One 15-ounce can tomato sauce
Juice of 1 orange
2 tablespoons smoked paprika
1 teaspoon ground ginger
¼ teaspoon nutmeg
¼ teaspoon allspice
½ teaspoon red pepper flakes
½ tablespoon molasses
2 teaspoons coconut aminos
Small splash/pinch of a sweetener of your choice
Optional: Celtic sea salt

PREPARATION:

1. In a small saucepan over low heat, warm the onion and garlic in olive oil for 1 minute. Add the tomato sauce and 1/2 can of water and stir until well-combined.

2. Stir in the orange juice, spices, pepper, molasses, coconut aminos, and sweetener of choice. Salt to taste.

3. Bring to a very slow simmer. Stir and allow to cook for 15 minutes or longer to thicken to your preference. Store in airtight jar in refrigerator.

Makes 12 ounces

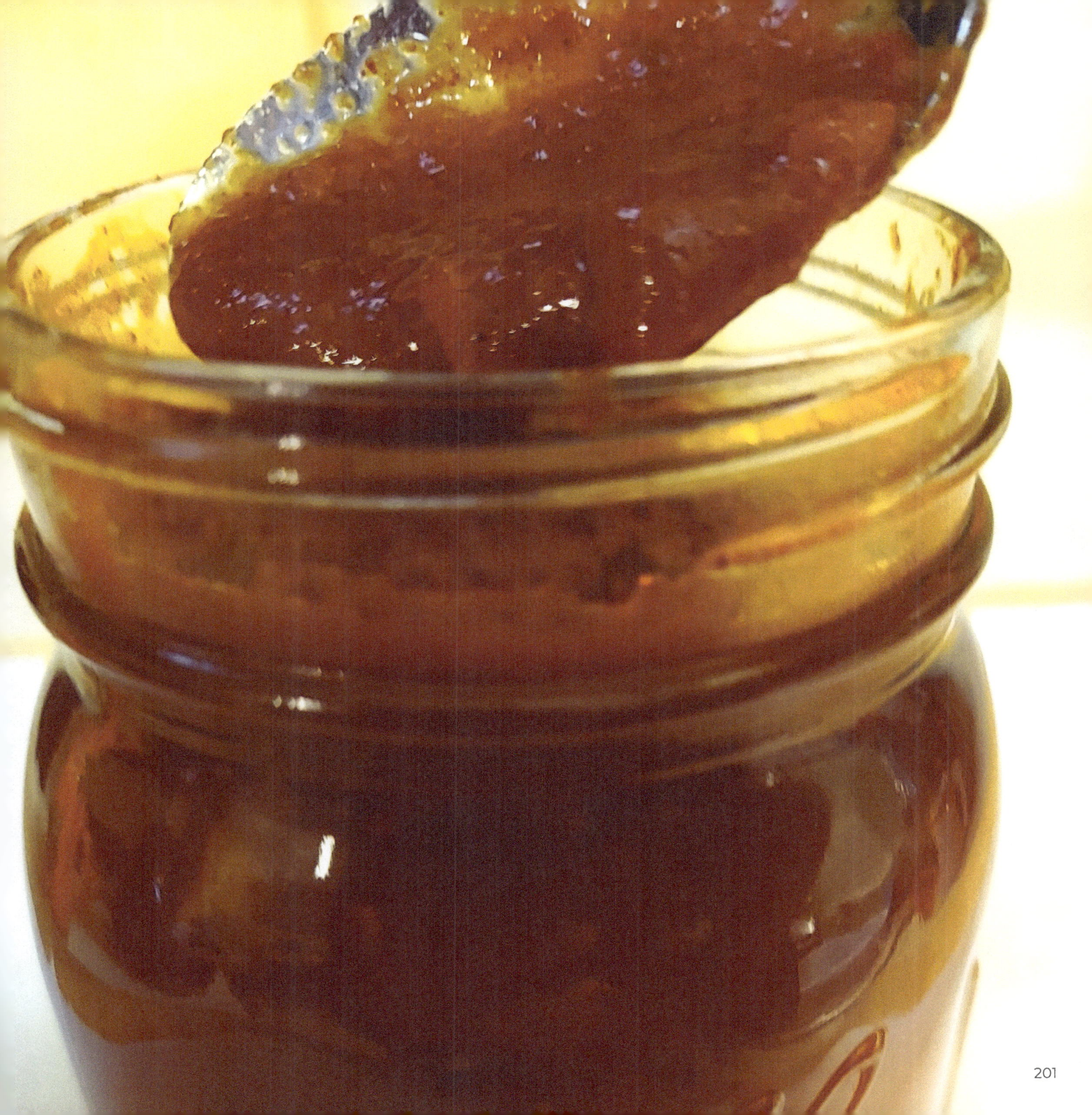

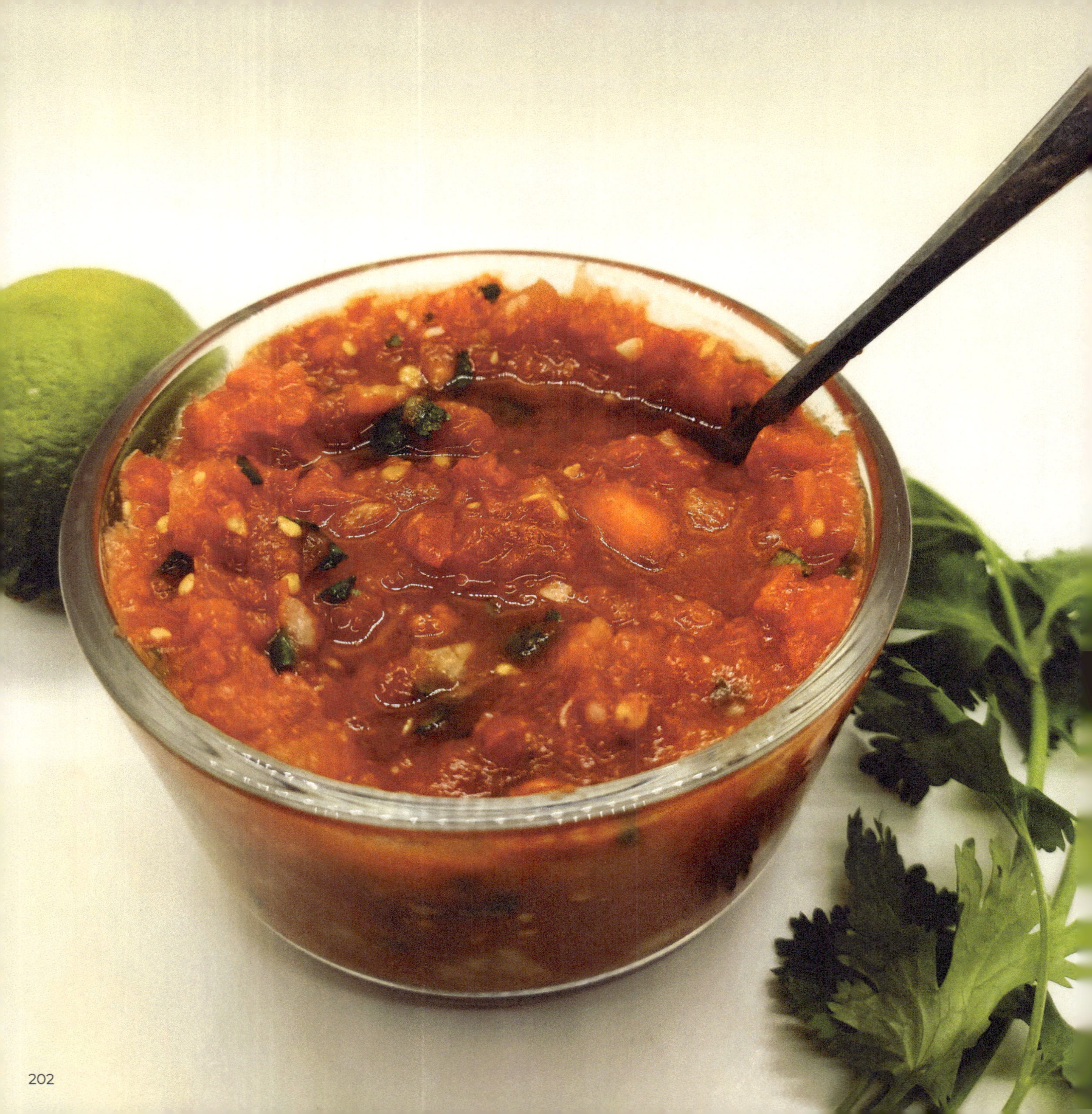

FRESH TOMATO SALSA

Salsa is especially good when the tomatoes are ripe. Mixing juicy tomatoes with flavors of lime, onions, cilantro and a little heat whether from peppers or spices is a delight. SO tasty, quick to prepare, fresh and refreshing.

INGREDIENTS:
2-3 fresh tomatoes, chopped
½ onion, chopped
Juice of lime
½ cup cilantro leaves, chopped
Salt and pepper to taste
Optional: chilies or jalapeno pepper

PREPARATION:

1. In a medium bowl, add tomatoes, lime juice and cilantro leaves. Blend ingredients together, taste and adjust flavors. Allow to stand for 15 minutes before serving for the flavors to intensify.

Makes 2 cups

DRESS THE SALAD

Whether you choose a light or creamy dressing for this vibrant salad both will be a hit. Hand crafted dressings give you control of the ingredients. The ingredients make all the difference!

Citrus- Turmeric Dressing

This dressing is light and fruity, the citrus sparkles while the mustard is a gentle lift for the beautiful bowl of peppers and the like.

INGREDIENTS:

Juice of orange
Juice of ½ lime
1/4 teaspoon ground turmeric
1/4 teaspoon ground ginger
1/2 teaspoon of whole grain mustard (page XX)
Salt and pepper to taste
Optional: sweetener if you chose

PREPARATION:

Whisk the ingredients together, taste and adjust to your palate or mood.

Makes 1 serving

Creamy Avocado Dressing

Here the avocado (fruit) is a healthy texture for spinach and blends well with the other veggies without being too heavy. There is nutrient richness in the avocado-spinach connection that is healthy for the heart.

INGREDIENTS:

1 avocado, pitted and cut into chunks
Juice of ½ lime
½ cup of non-dairy milk
¼ teaspoon onion powder
½ teaspoon Celtic sea salt or not
Optional: Hand full of parsley leaves

PREPARATION:

Put all ingredients in a blender and blend until smooth. Taste and adjust to your desired taste. Add water for a thinner dressing. Store in air tight container in the refrigerator up to 2 weeks.

Makes 1 serving

Sesame Seed Sprinkles

Calcium and magnesium rich. Mixed with a little ground ginger for taste and seasoning. In Japan, Gomasi is a condiment of black and tan sesame seeds and salt, said to be used in place of salt.

INGREDIENTS:

½ cup tan sesame seeds
½ cup black sesame seeds
½ tablespoon ground ginger

PREPARATION:

Combine ingredients, adjust ingredients your liking. Store in an airtight container.

Makes 1 cup

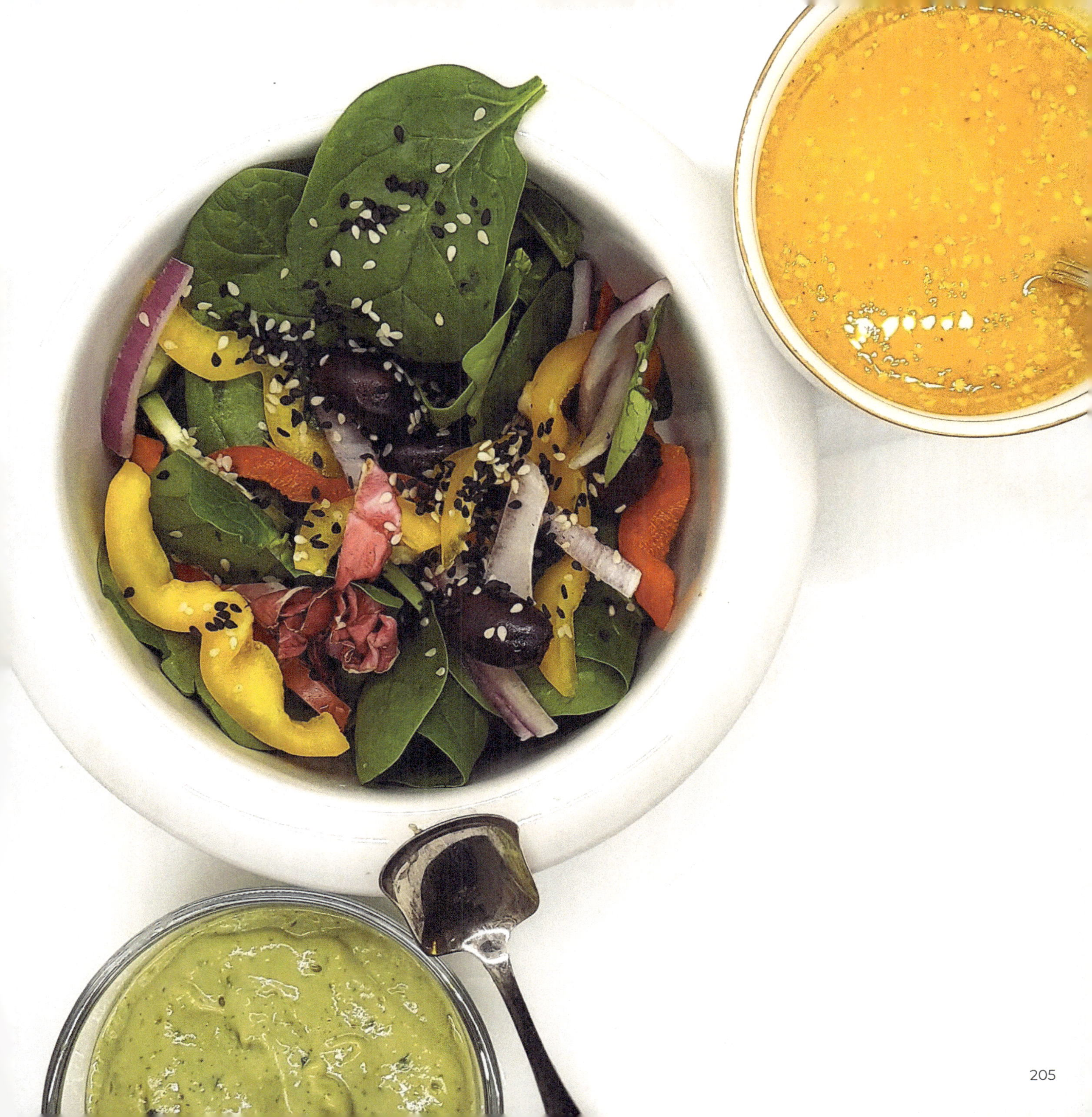

Beverages - Desserts Vegetables and Fruit

(partial listing)

Swiss Chard

Zucchini

Apple (Green, Red)

Avocado

Banana

Black berries

Blueberries

Celery

Kiwi

Lemons

Lime

Oranges

Pomegranate

Raspberries

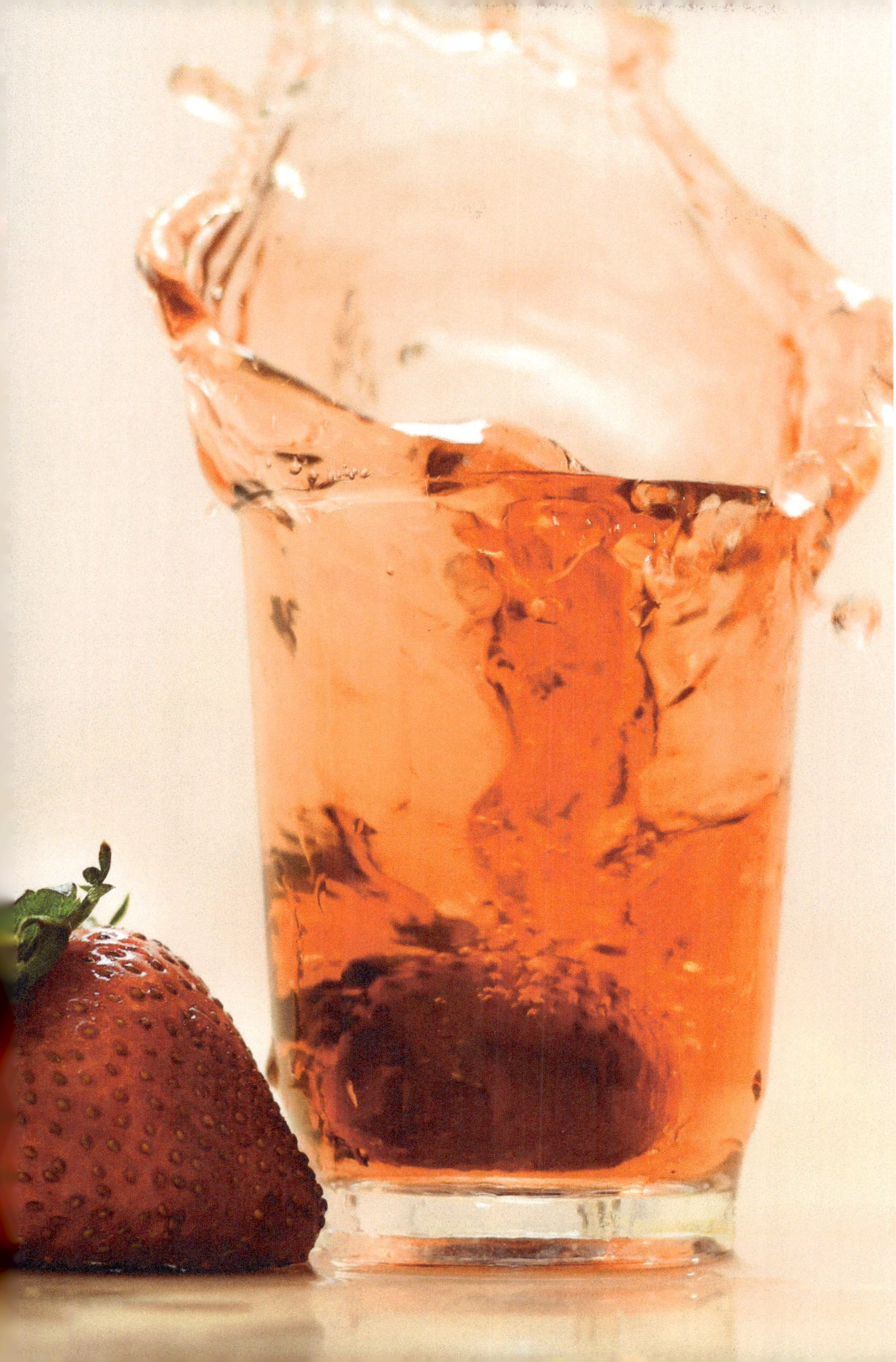

BEVERAGES AND DESSERTS

RECIPES FOR BEVERAGES AND DESSERTS

Beverages and desserts certainly have a prominent place in plant-based eating and lifestyle. These are areas that tantalize our taste buds. Most traditional beverages and desserts are full of refined carb, unhealthy fats and loads of sugar. The good news is as you re-define your relationship to food, you will discover many tasty, nutritious options available in every phrase of your new food experience. Take the time to be a conscience consumer. Reading and understanding product labels is an important habit to cultivate (see Understanding Food Labels). Be aware of foods that will hinder your ability to succeed at reaching your health goals, whether your goal is: weight loss, coming off medication or just being fully mobile, alert and in best health.

Be encouraged to drink at least eight glasses of water daily to stay hydrated and to improve your physical performance. In the recipes that follow I have incorporated fruit, flowers, vegetables, herbs, and spices into beverages and desserts with as little sweetener and unhealthy fats as possible. Have fun in the kitchen!

Let's Welcome Beverages and Desserts!

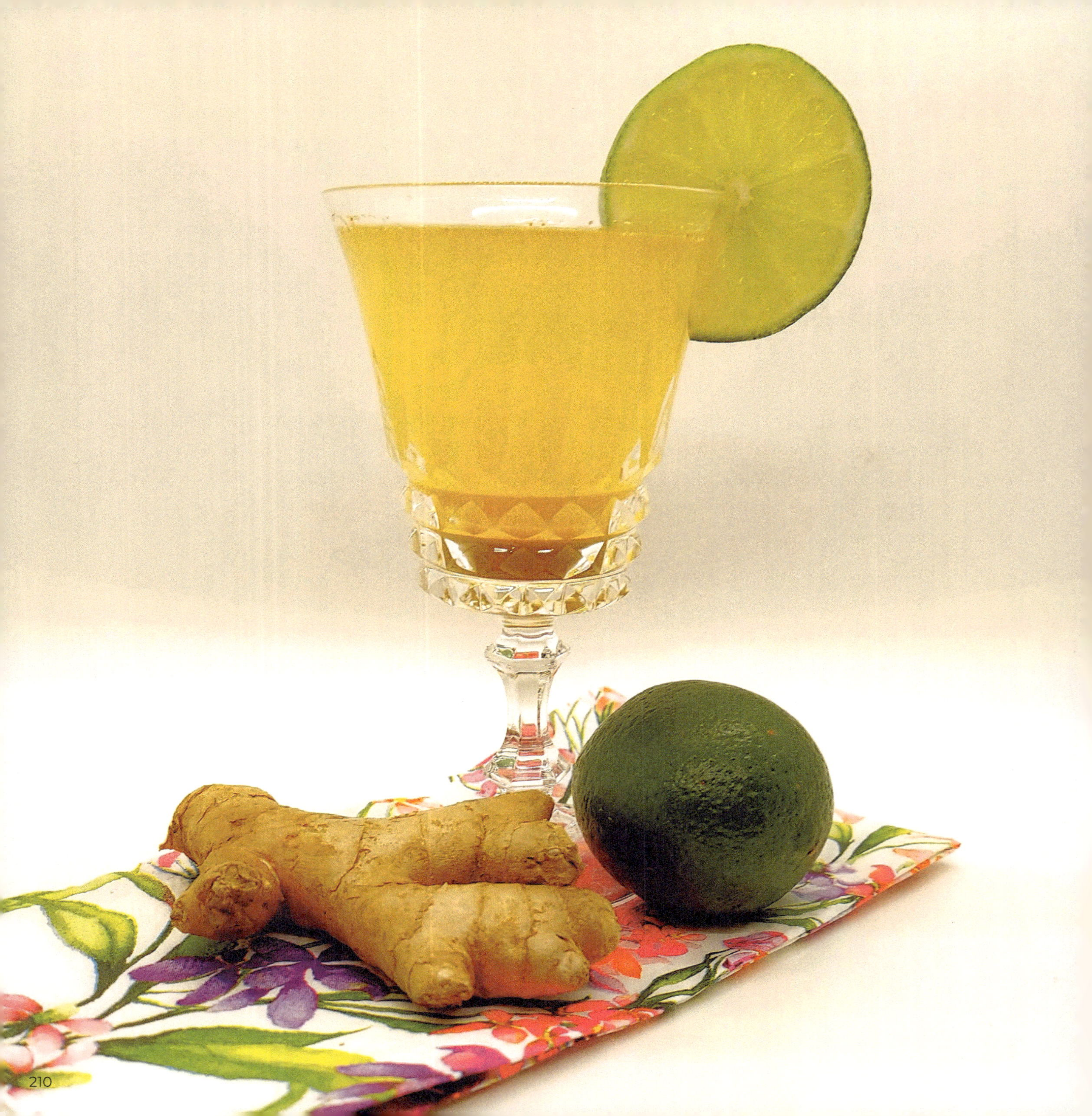

LIME-GINGERADE

Limes are high in Vitamin C, which boost the immune system and aid in digestion. Since ancient times, ginger has also been known for its anti-inflammatory properties. Together, lime and ginger are a powerful team!

INGREDIENTS:
1½ teaspoons ground ginger
Juice of 1 lime (3 tablespoons)
Optional: Sweetener of your choice

PREPARATION:

1. Spoon the ground ginger into a glass and pour the lime juice over it. Add 2 cups of chilled water and stir well. Taste and add sweetener as you like.

2. This makes a strong drink! You can add more water to soften its flavor

Makes 2 cups

HIBISCUS TEA

Hibiscus (sorrel) flowers make a nutritious drink enjoyed in many parts of the world under different names. Sorrel drink, Zobo beverage and Aqua de Jamacia all refer to hibiscus tea. Each culture infuses its own unique spice blends into this tart flavored tea. It is loaded with Vitamin C, antioxidants and contains amazing health benefits. Come drink to your health.

INGREDIENTS:
6 cups of water
1/2 cup dried hibiscus flowers
1 cinnamon stick
5 whole cloves
Maple syrup (sweeten to taste)
Options: splash lime juice, a sprig of mint (garnish)

PREPARATION:

1. Add water to a medium saucepan and bring to a boil. Cut the heat off. Stir in the dried flowers and whole spices. Cover, remove from heat and let stand (steep)for 30 minutes.

2. Pour through a strainer into a glass container and sweeten to taste. If too strong, dilute with water. Serve cold, with a splash of line and sprig of mint (optional)

Makes 1 Quart (32 ounces)

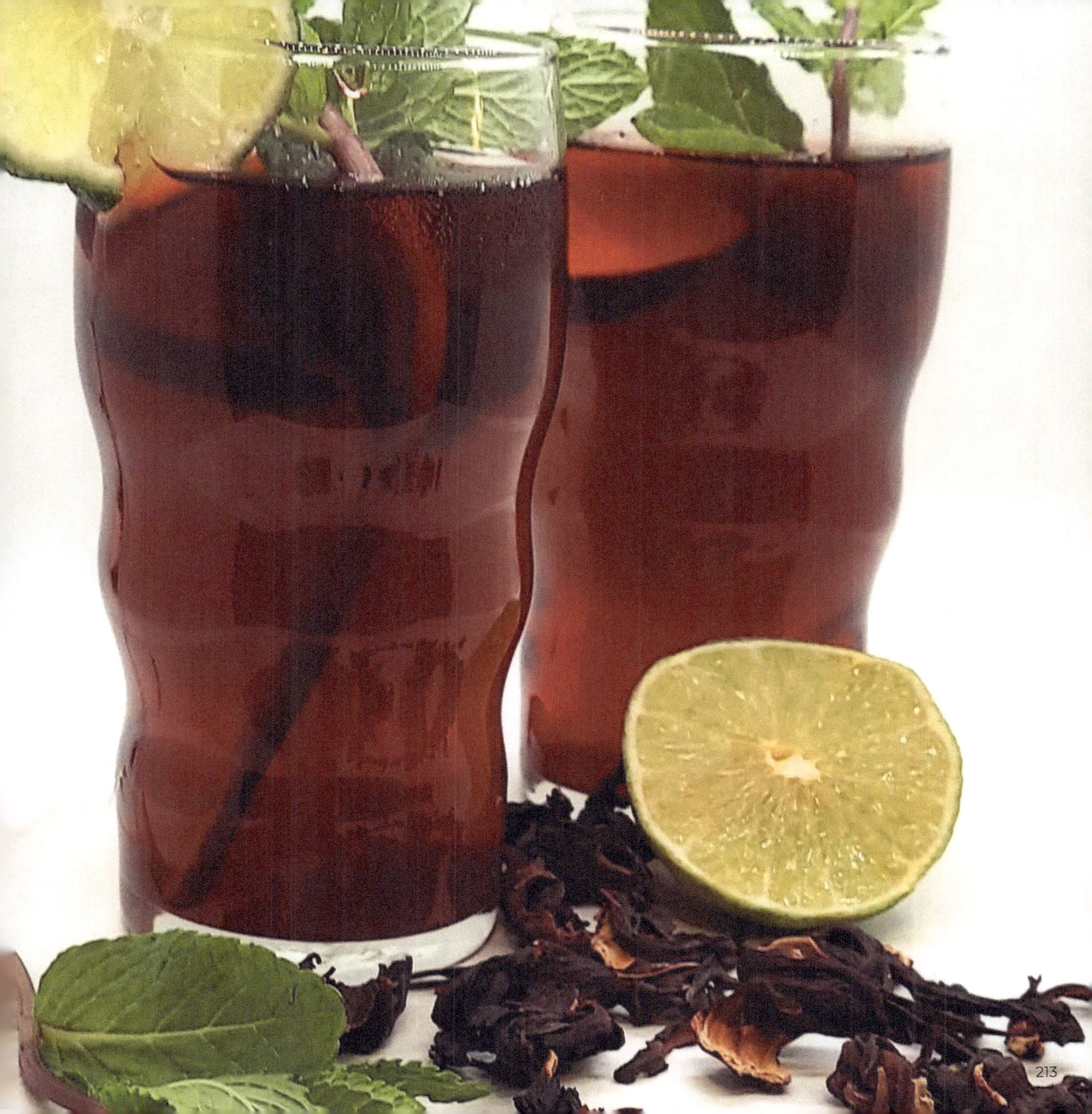

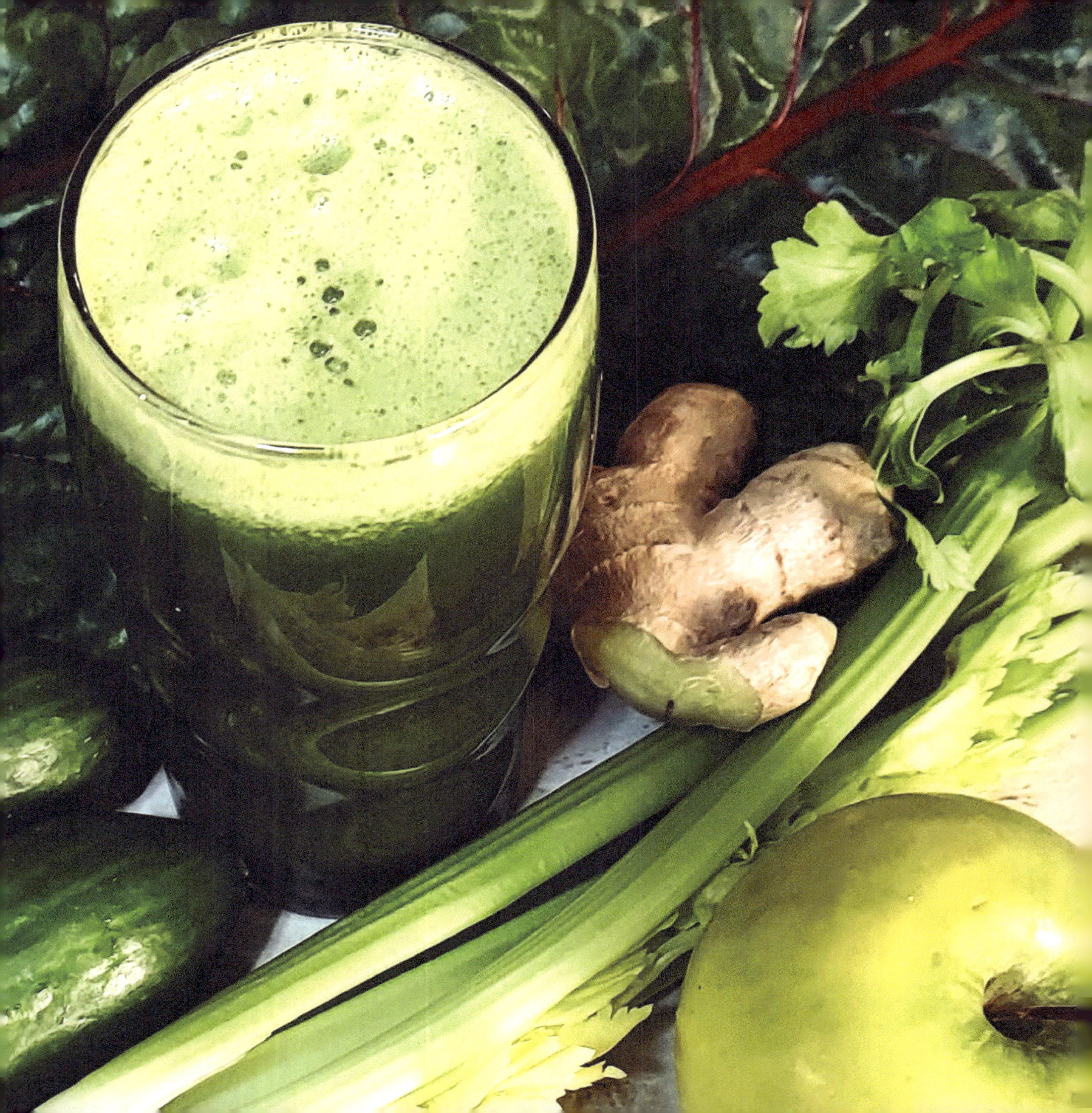

GREEN JUICE

Allow this recipe to be a template for you. Choose a leafy green- your source of chlorophyll, add another green vegetable, then a fruit that juice can be extracted from and ginger as a great flavor enhancer. Use organics vegetables when juicing.

INGREDIENTS:

4 large Swiss chard leaves (or leafy green of your choice)
1 green apple cut in quarters
1 zucchini, cut in chucks
1 rib celery, cut
1 inch ginger root, skin off and cut in half

PREPARATION:

Wash and dry vegetables. Feed each item into the juicer (extractor). Taste and enjoy!

Makes 6-8 ounces

ORANGE ALMOND SMOOTHIE

The almonds in this drink are the protein, cashew butter / milk may also be used. Oranges add the vitamin C and come in a variety, pick your favorite. Flax or chia seed for Omega 3. Bananas as a sweetener, frozen bananas make the smoothie icy.

INGREDIENTS:
1 cup almond milk
2 tablespoons almond butter (or 24 raw almonds)
2 oranges (peeled and segmented)
1 banana (frozen is best) in chunks
1 tablespoon chia seeds (or ground flax seeds)

PREPARATION:

1. Place each item into a high-speed blender or nutri-bullet and blend until smooth. You can adjust the thickness of the smoothie by adding additional milk, or water.

Makes 2 servings

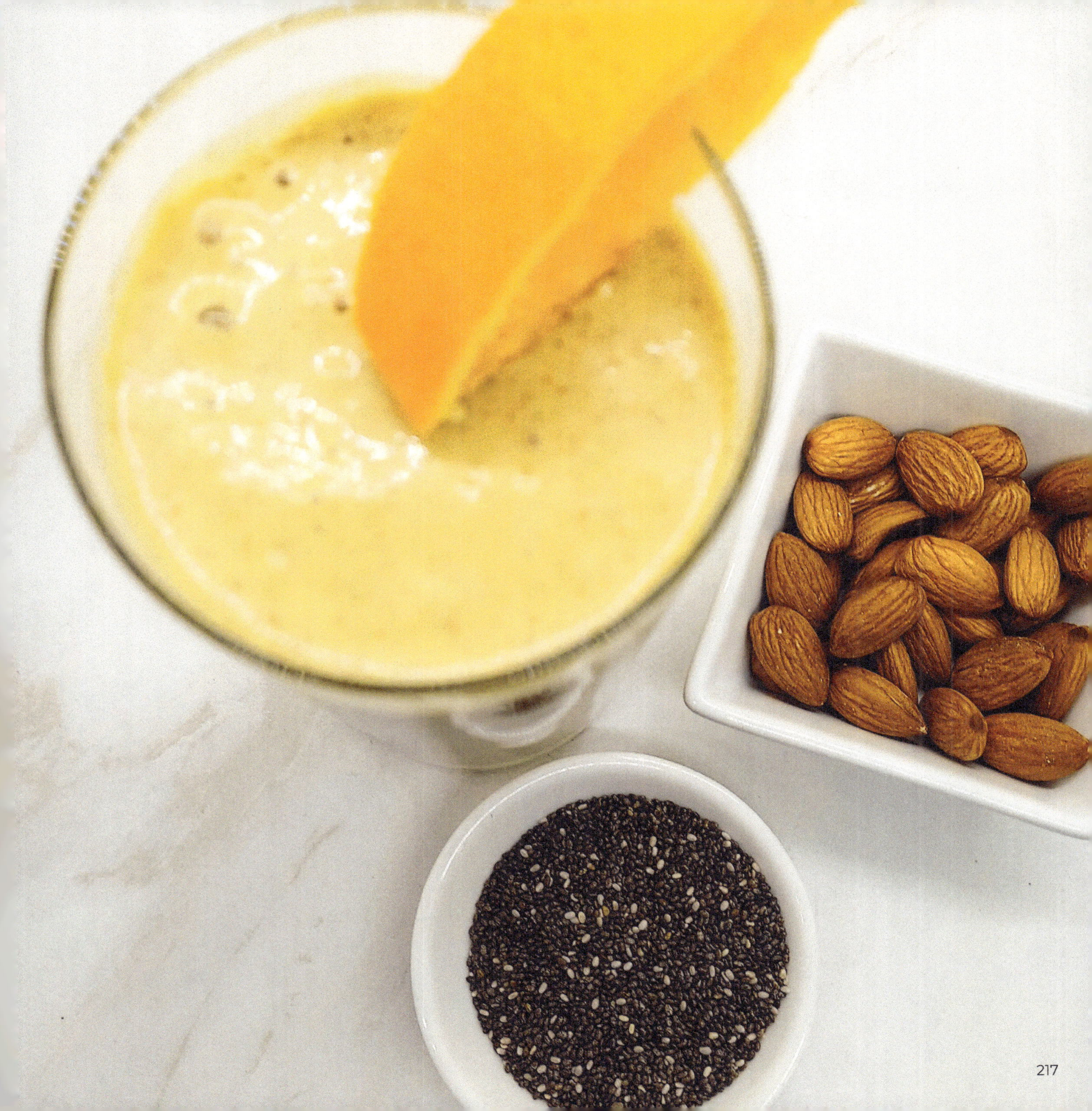

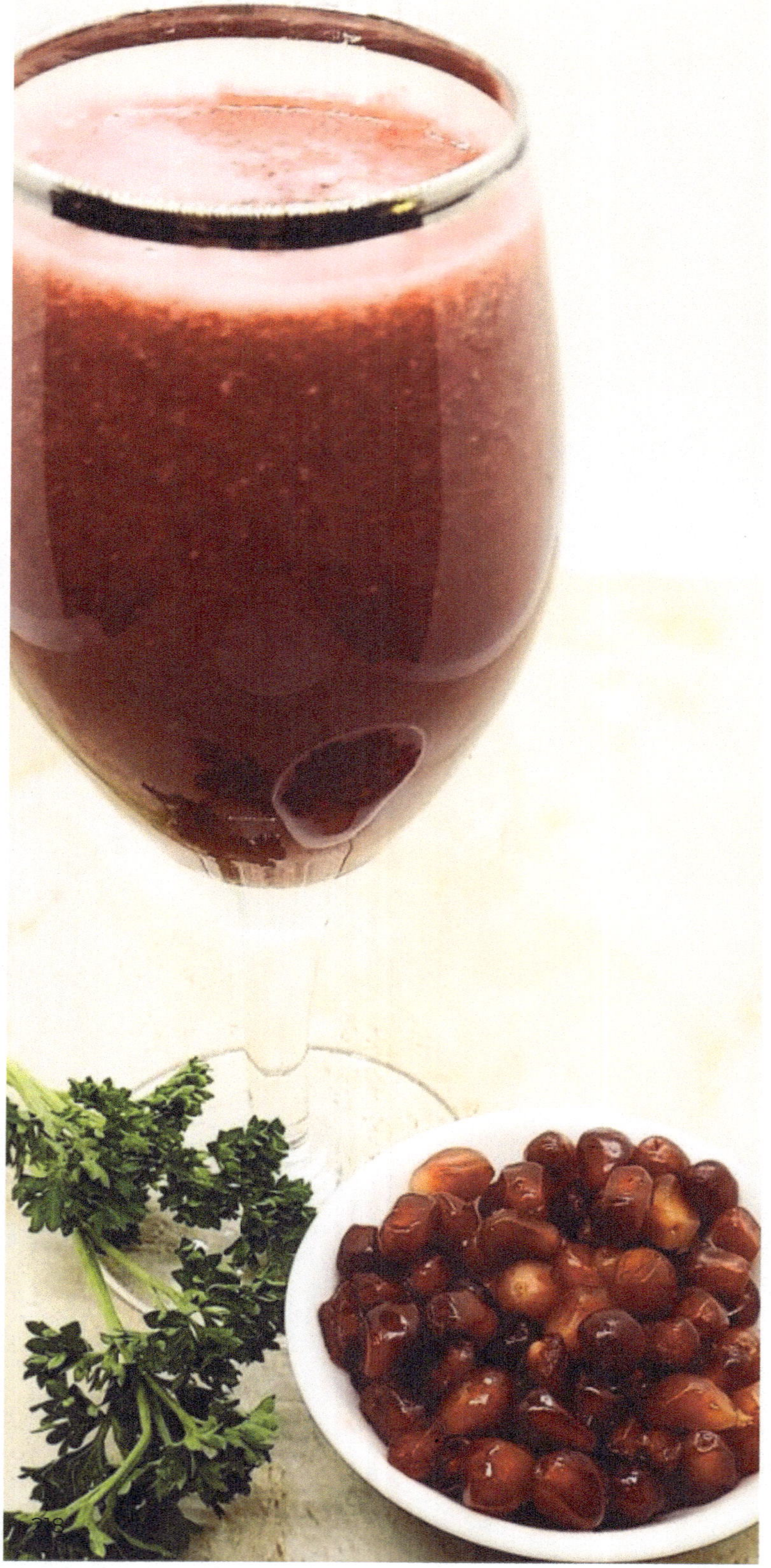

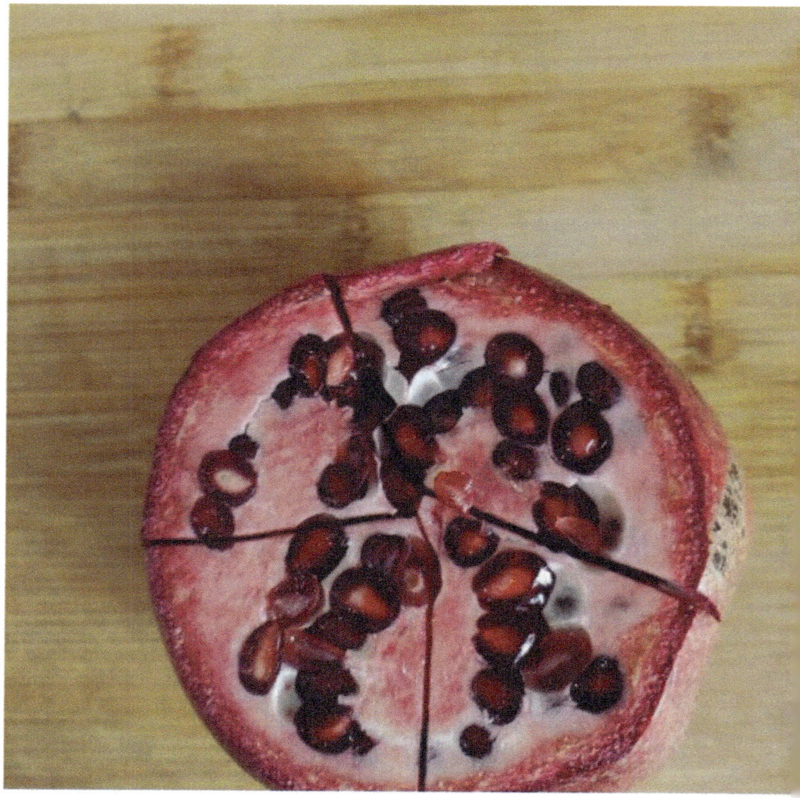

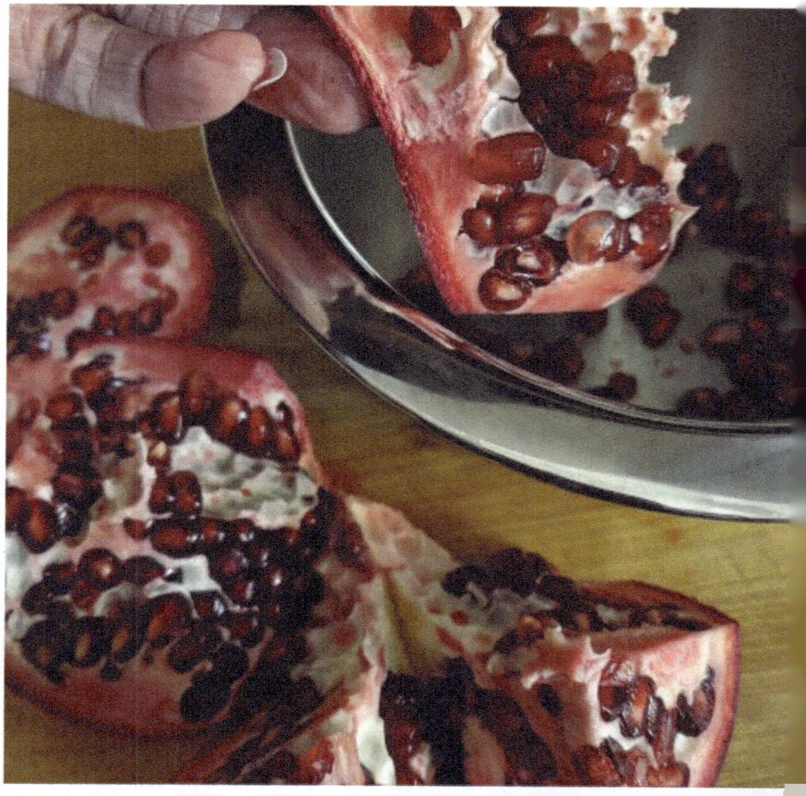

POMEGRANATE JUICE

Pomegranates are a "super food". The arils (seeds) in the pomegranate are rich in antioxidants and are a great source of vitamin A, C, and E. They are also cancer fighters, an aid for fatigue and lost energy and have anti-aging properties. Pomegranate arils can also be purchased individually.

INGREDIENTS:
Arils (seeds) of 2 pomegranates

PREPARATION:

1. Place pomegranate seeds in a blender and pulse. Pour through a strainer, mash with the back of a spoon, press out all of the juice.

2. Pour the pomegranate juice into pitcher or glass, to drink straight or add 1/4 cup water. Stir and drink.

Makes 2 servings

HOW TO DE-SEED A POMEGRANATE

Remove the arils (seeds) from the pomegranate by first slicing the top of the pomegranate and making a smooth surface. Many people remove the arils under water (in a large bowl with water) so all splashing from the seeds is under the water.

Score through the white membrane as in the photo. Pull the sections apart and gently brush the seeds loose into the bowl, whether under water or into a bowl without water. You can also turn pomegranate upside down and with a spoon gently knock the arils loose.

Pull apart one section at a time until the entire pomegranate has been de-seeded. Then repeat with second pomegranate.

RUBY WINTER ORANGE DRINK

This citrus drink is full of fiber, potassium, and vitamin C. It is good to you and for you. Blood oranges, a winter fruit, are usually readily available around the winter holidays.

INGREDIENTS:
Juice of ½ lime
Juice of 1 orange
Juice of 1 blood orange
1 banana in chunks (frozen is best)
Handful of blueberries or blackberries

PREPARATION:

1. Pour the juices into the blender, add the banana and berries followed by 3 cups of water

2. Blend well. If the bananas are not frozen, enjoy over ice.

Makes 2 cups

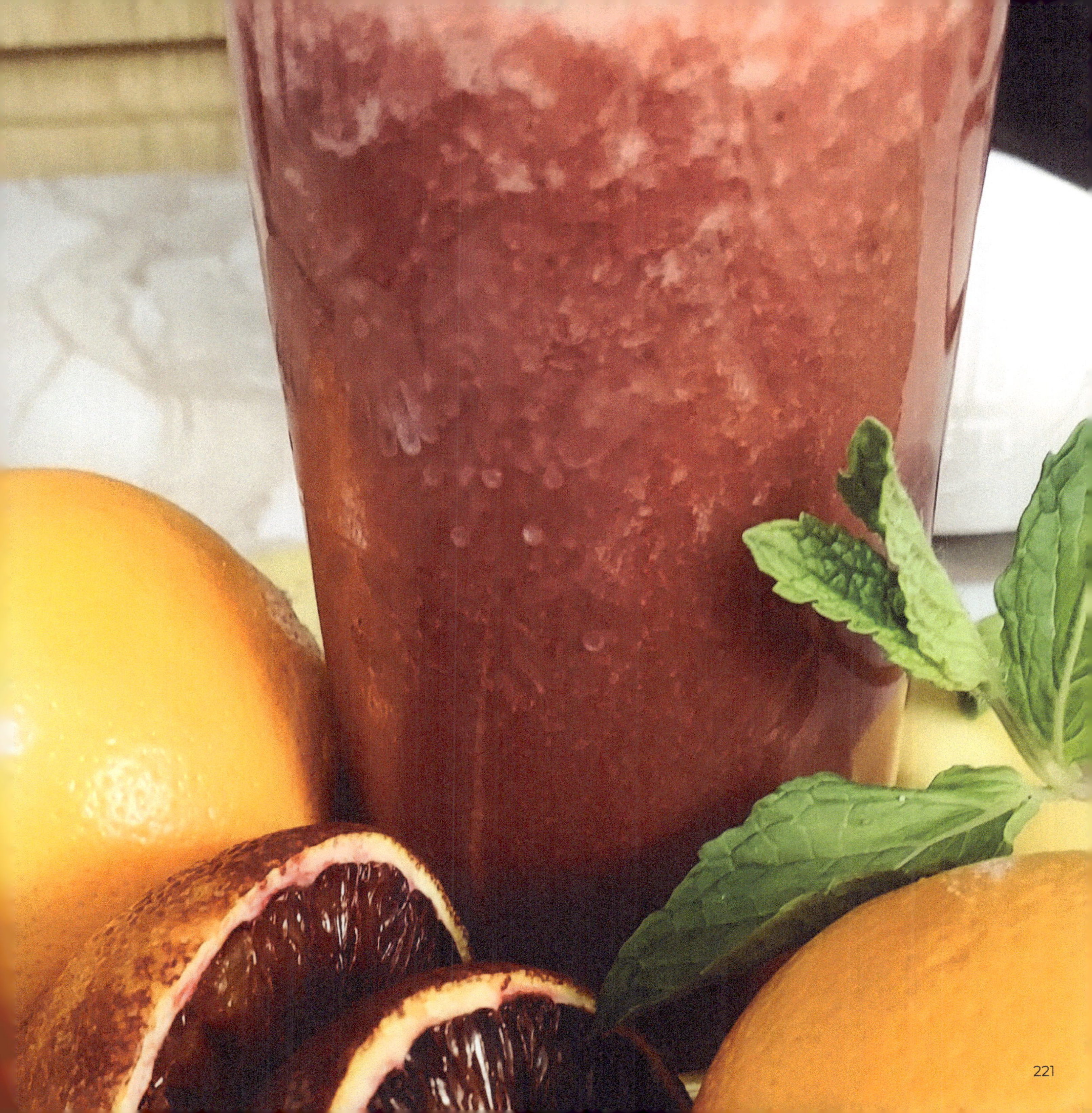

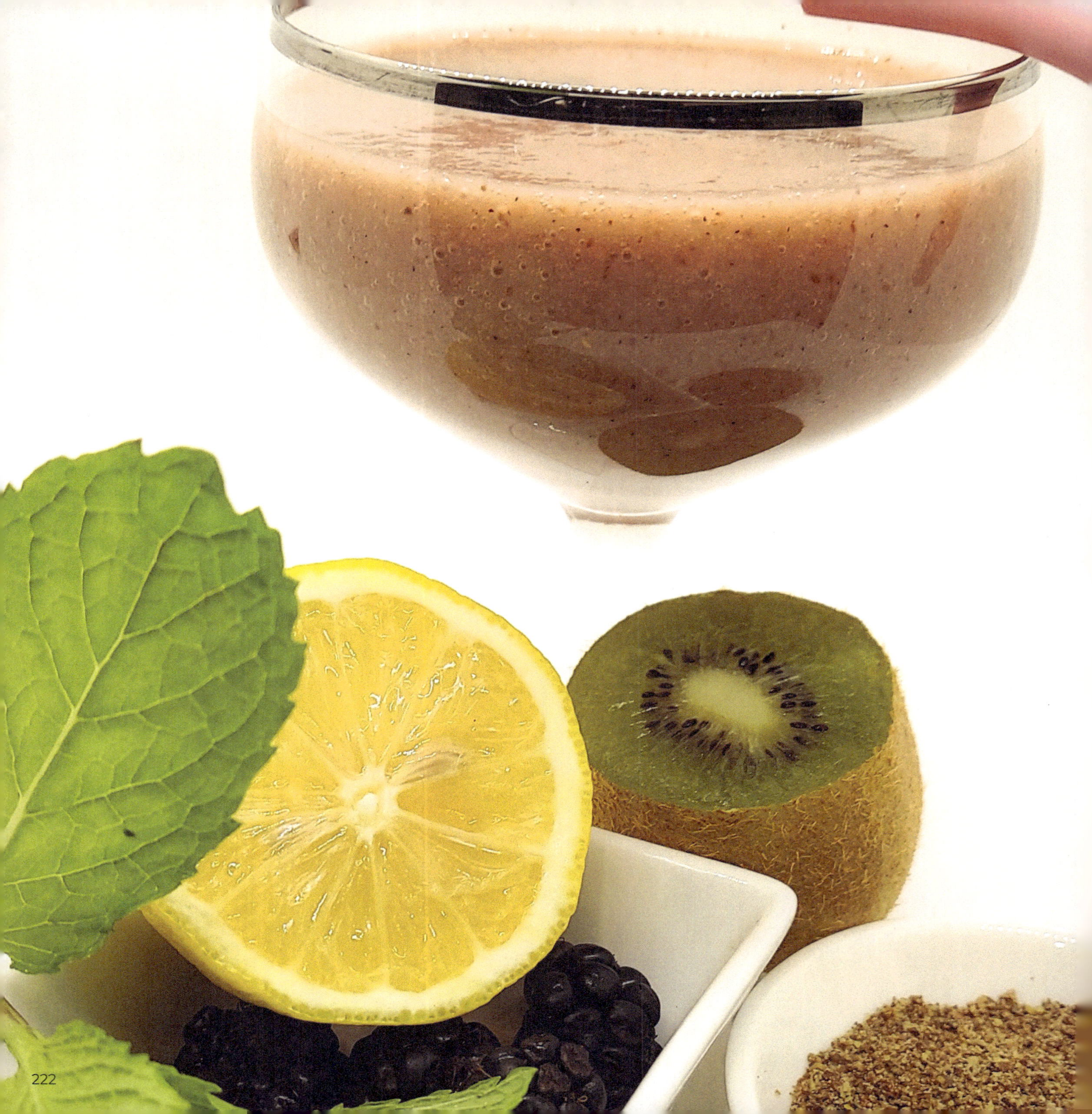

KIWI-BERRY SMOOTHIE

Kiwi is vitamin C rich, frozen banana chunks alleviate need for ice cubes. The berries add an anti-aging property and the flax seeds supply omega 3.

INGREDIENTS:

1 kiwi, skin removed
4 blackberries
1 frozen banana, (in chunks)
¼ teaspoon ginger
Juice of ½ lemon
1 tablespoon ground flax seeds (or hemp seeds)

PREPARATION:

Place all ingredients in a blender along with ½ cup of water and blend well.

Makes 12 ounces

SPRING BERRY CRUMBLE

This crumble is a quick and fun anytime treat. Blackberries , blueberries, and raspberries lead the way seasonally and are high in antioxidants. The phytonutrient anthocyanin is the blue, red and violet hue in the berries. Berries are good for the heart, promote anti-aging and healthy tissue growth.

INGREDIENTS:
1 teaspoon ground cinnamon
½ teaspoon ground nutmeg
2 tablespoons fresh lemon juice
1 teaspoon vanilla extract
3 tablespoons agave nectar
1 tablespoon arrowroot powder
3 cups raspberries, blackberries, and/or blueberries, washed and well-drained

Crumble Topping:
½ cup walnuts
¼ cup spelt flour
½ cup rolled oats
½ cup coconut sugar
1 teaspoon ground cinnamon
¼ teaspoon Celtic sea salt
3 tablespoons coconut oil, plus extra for the pan

PREPARATION: Preheat oven to 375°F. Oil a Pyrex 9"x 5" loaf pan.

1. In a small bowl, mix together the spices, lemon juice, vanilla extract, and agave nectar. Add the arrowroot powder and blend well.

2. Add the well-drained berries to the oiled pan. Pour the arrowroot mixture over the berries and mix gently.

CRUMBLE TOPPING:

3. In a small food processor, grind the walnuts to a pebble-like consistency, then place in a bowl. Add the spelt flour, oats, coconut sugar, cinnamon, and salt.

4. Using a fork or pastry blender, blend the coconut oil into the crumble. Sprinkle the crumble topping evenly over the berry mixture.

5. Place on a cookie sheet and bake until berries are bubbling, approximately 30 minutes. Let cool, then serve and enjoy!

Makes 4 to 6 servings

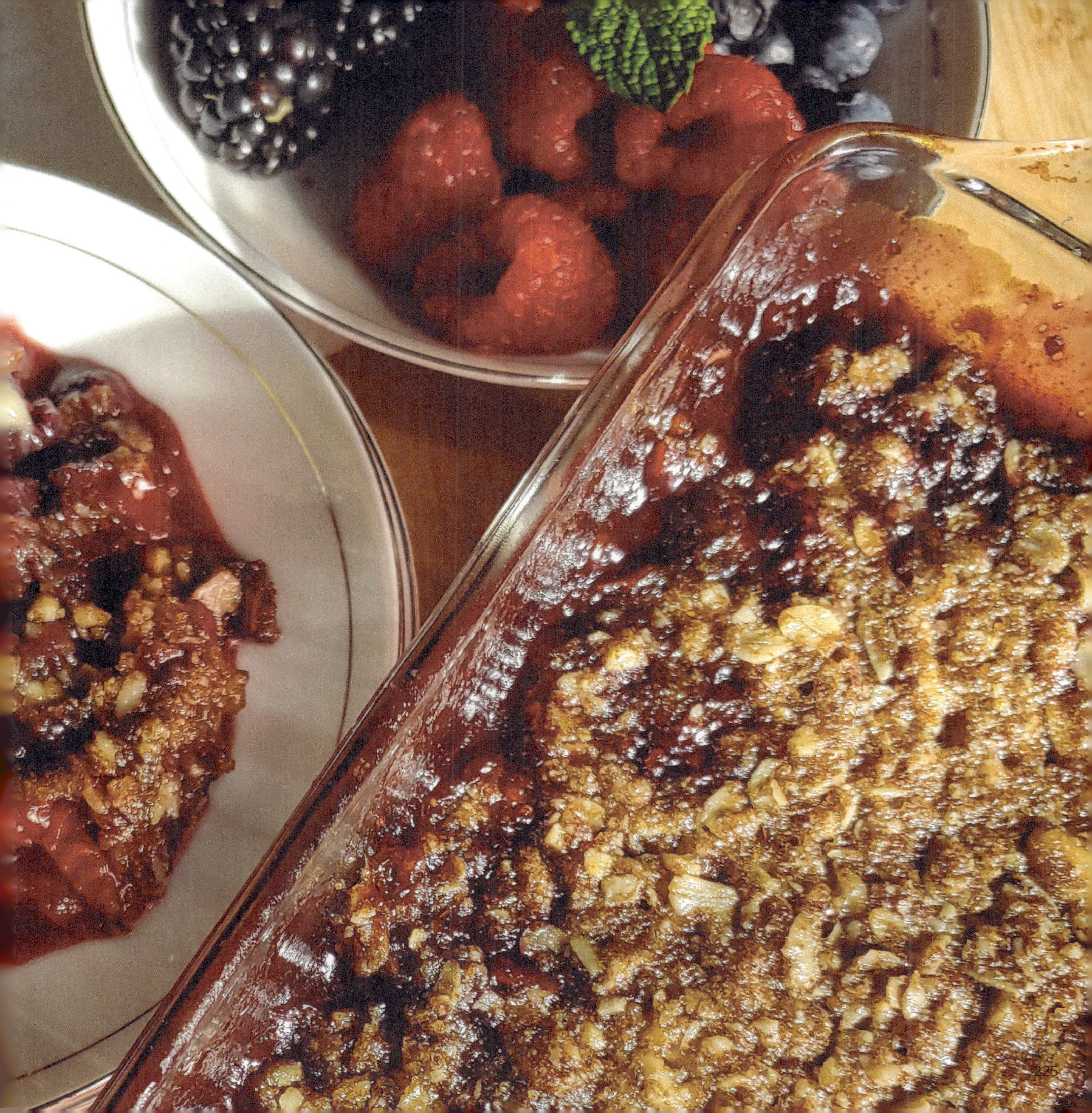

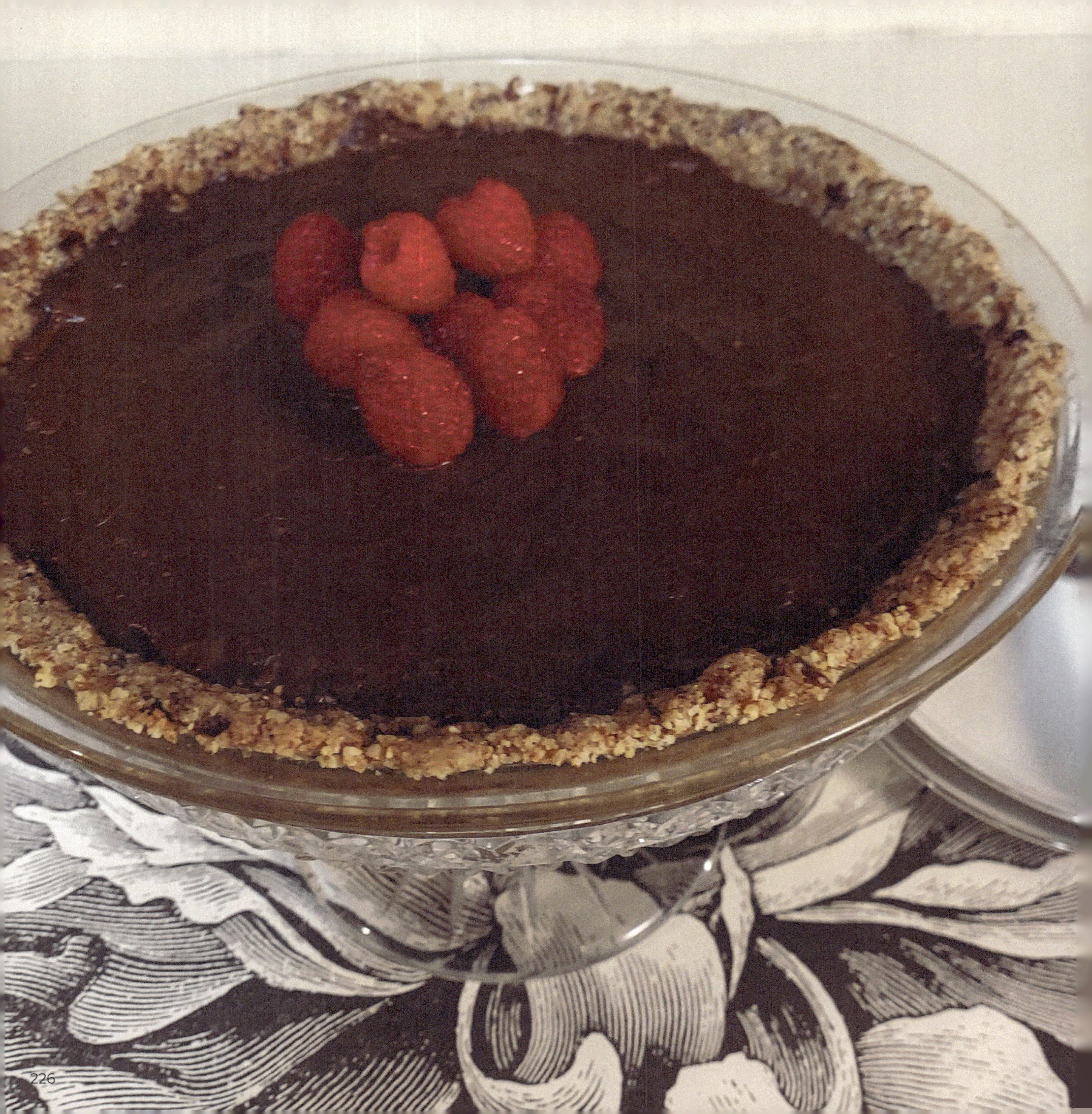

CACAO AVOCADO PIE IN WALNUT CRUST

Avocado is a fruit loaded with good fat which is combined with cacao powder, the pure form of chocolate. The result is a highly nutrient-dense pie. These super foods are sitting in walnuts the perfect brain food. How cool is that!

INGREDIENTS:
3 ripe avocados
1 teaspoon balsamic vinegar
2 teaspoons vanilla extract
1/2 cup cacao powder (Theobroma, preferred)
½ cup maple syrup
1 tablespoon coconut oil

Walnut- Almond Crust
1-1/2 cups raw walnuts
1 cup pitted dates (10) If dates are dry, soak in ½ cup filtered water 10 minutes.
½ teaspoon vanilla extract

PREPARATION: Lightly oil 9.5" pie pan

1. Put walnuts into blender and pulse a couple times. Add vanilla, and 3-4 dates at a time. Pulse until dates are blended with the nuts

2. Pour nut mixture onto pie pan and press mixture firmly into pie pan forming an even layer of crust. Place in freezer to firm at least 30 minutes.

3. Prepare the filling: place avocados, balsamic, vanilla, cacao powder, sweetener and oil into a high power blender and blend until smooth.

4. Remove pie crust from the freezer and scoop the cacao filling into the shell. Distribute the filling evenly and return to the freezer for at least an hour. Remove 30 minutes before serving.

Makes 4 to 6 servings

COCONUT CREAM WITH FRUIT

When you may want just a taste of sweetness at the end of a meal. This whipped coconut cream is light and refreshing. Top with your choice of soften fruit, or compote, with a drizzle of maple syrup. Coconut cream alone makes a great topping for Cacao Hot Chocolate (page 180)

INGREDIENTS:
I- 14 oz can of full fat coconut cream, refrigerated overnight, it must be cold.

Options: Cinnamon and/or vanilla to mix into the cream for added flavor
Topping in picture. Blueberry compote (page 184)

NOTE: Refrigerate at least 12 hours. This allows the liquid and cream to separate.

PREPARATION:

1. Open the can, scoop the harden coconut cream into a bowl. Save the liquid (add to smoothies, etc.)

2. Using an electric mixer, blend the cream gently until the cream is firm and fluffy. Top with your choice of fruit, coconut, finely ground nuts, etc.

Makes 2 cups

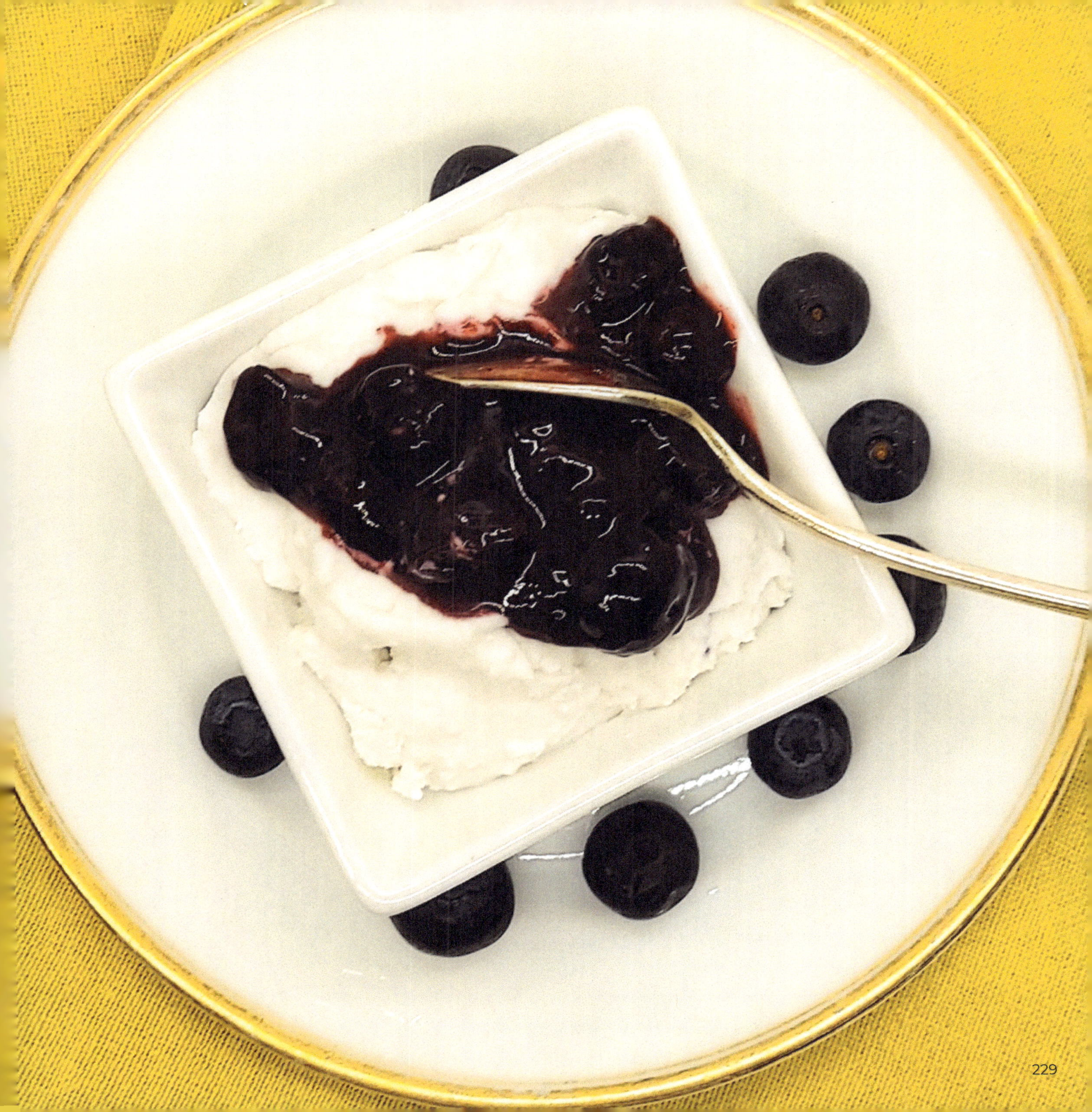

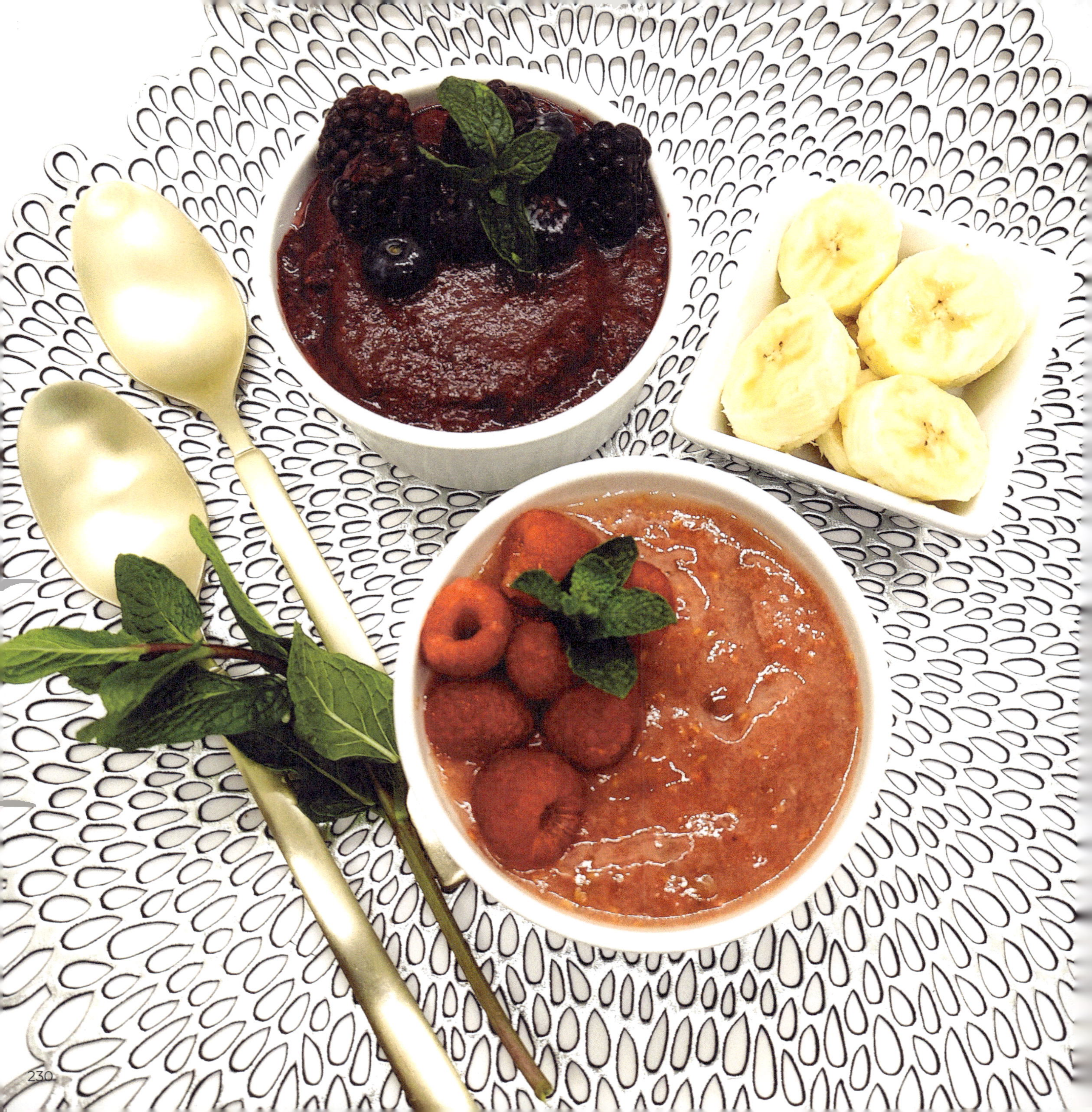

RASPBERRY BANANA (ICE) CREAM

Frozen banana chunks are a handy item to have on hand in the freezer. I use them in my smoothies and for a quick dessert idea like this. Raspberries, blueberries, and other (low sugar) fruit that is on hand will make a delicious, quick icy cream blend.

INGREDIENTS:
1 pint of raspberries
2 bananas, in chunks

PREPARATION:

1. Using a high-speed bender or nutri-bullet, combine ingredients. Pulse the mixture on low – to- medium first then scrape sides and continue until all is blended.

2. Transfer to a freezer safe container and place in freezer for at least 2 hours. Can store in the freezer for up to 1 week.

Makes 1 serving

APPLE WALNUT OATMEAL COOKIE

This oatmeal cookie is a vegan sweet treat. Apples, walnuts, and warm spices bring it to life. Grated carrots are also a great substitute for the apples.

INGREDIENTS:
1 cup spelt flour
1 cup rolled oats
1 teaspoon aluminum free baking powder
½ teaspoon baking soda
1 teaspoon ground cinnamon
½ teaspoon ground ginger
¼ teaspoon ground nutmeg
¼ cup coconut sugar
¼ teaspoon Celtic sea salt
2/3 cups chopped walnuts
1 apple grated (1 cup)
1/3 cup coconut oil (warmed)
¼ cup maple syrup

PREPARATION: Pre-heat oven 350°F.

1. In a large bowl add flour, oats, baking powder baking soda, spices, sugar and salt. Blend in apples and walnuts. In a separate bowl add the coconut oil and maple syrup.
2. Add the wet ingredients to the flour mixture and stir just to combine. On a parchment lined baking sheet, place portions of cookie dough, well-spaced apart. Bake for 12-15 minutes or until cookies are golden on top and bottom.
3. Remove from the oven and allow to cool. Store in a sealed container up to a week.

Makes 6 large, 1 dozen medium, or 16 small cookies

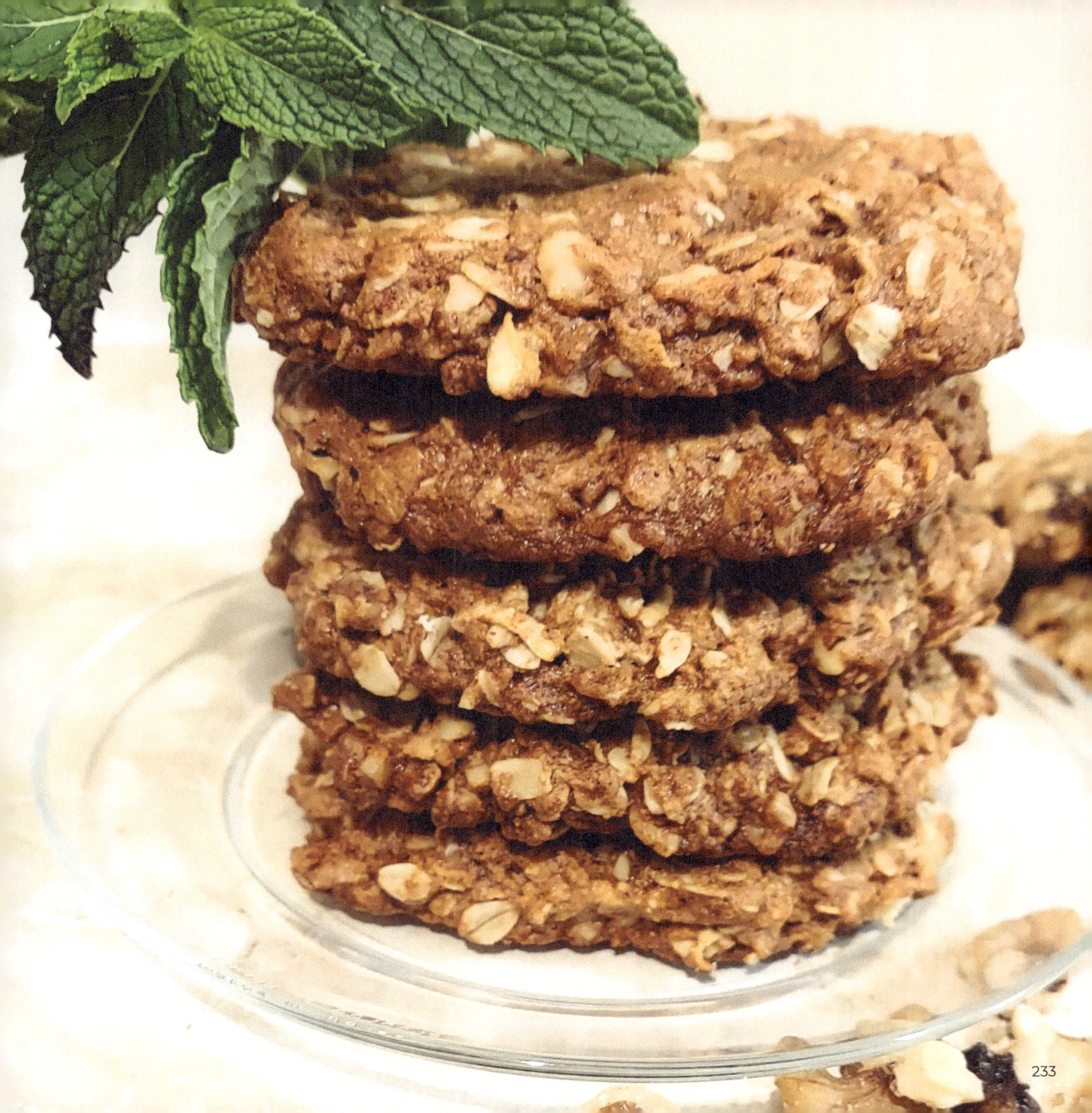

EQUIVALENT MEASUREMENTS

Unit	Equals	Also equals	Produce	Pounds
1 teaspoon	1/6 fl. oz.	1/3 tablespoon		
1 tablespoon	½ fl. oz.	3 teaspoons		
1/8 cup	1 fl. oz.	2 tablespoons		
		3 tablespoons	1 lime-lemon (juiced)	
¼ cup	2 fl. Oz	4 tablespoons		
1/3 cup	2 ¾ fl. oz.	¼ cup + 4 teaspoons		
½ cup	4 fl. oz.	8 tablespoons	Small Onion	¼ lb.
1 cup	8 fl. oz.	½ pint	Medium Onion	½ lb.
	12 fl. Oz.	1-1/2 cups	Large Onion	
1 pint	16 fl. oz.	2 cups		1 lb.
1 quart	32 fl. oz.	2 pints		2 lbs.
1 liter	34 fl. oz	1 quart + ¼ cup		
1 gallon	128 fl. oz.	4 quarts		8 lbs.

ACKNOWLEDGEMENTS

My deepest gratitude to The Lord, my God for the assignment. Without that gentle nudging it may not have happened. I worked at Conte Nast publications and Doubleday and Co. in New York City at eighteen years of age. I believed then that one day I would pen a book, but a cookbook...

As things were changing, I realized truths that reside in me and was summoned to add my two cents. It has been such a journey.

Thank you to my family, Ayanna, Hajj, Kasandra, Kennedy for support all the way through.

Hajj for never giving up on this project, for the Art direction and cover design.

Michele Tate for beautifully bringing the cover design to life and the interior to completion. I am so very grateful.

Thank you to Dr. Kathleen Gregg, Dr. Joel Kahn, Dr. Akua Woolbright, Don Cinzori and Erin Beattie for believing in this work, endorsing, and encouraging me to keep it moving.

Thank you to Lisa Howard for her editorial services, patience, and diligence with the manuscript.

Suzette Carter Saulnier for proofreading and being available to help me sort out the structure. Maxine Shawver for editing and shaping the flow from recipe to recipe.

I am very grateful for all recipe testers, starting with my first proofreader and recipe tester my sister, Sharon Piper, niece Bareka Allen and Mary Fuglaar. My greatest cheerleader at the time 4-year-old Kennedy Nicole in the kitchen with me and my niece Rukiya Higgins encouraging me to get the book out.

Special Thanks to Doris Hayes, Sonda Miller, Dee Sandel and Deborah. These women cook for real, who tested, wrote comments, and inspired me to be a better cook, and appreciate the life of professional cooks, chefs, home cooks.

A heart of gratitude to all my dear friends for believing in me, praying with and for me; Including Michele January, Robin Mooney, Crescendi Mickens, Serene Gooden, Beverly Cage-Cooper, Patricia Saddler, and more. Praise the Lord for all who benefit from this cookbook.

REFERENCES

FOOD SELECTION – FOOD STORAGE

Page 22: https://www.fda.gov/food/food-labeling-nutrition/organic-food-labels

Page 26: https://foodrevolution.org/blog/eating-the-rainbow-health-benefits/

Page 21: https://foodrevolution.org/blog/eating-the-rainbow-health-benefits/

Page 35: https://foodsandfit.com/foods-not-to-put-in-the-fridge/

Page 38: https://foodsandfit.com/how-to-save-space-in-the-freezer/

Page 44: http://www.cliffordawright.com/caw/food/entries/display.php/topic_id/6/id/103/

RECIPES

Page 54: https://www.almanac.com/news/home-health/natural-living/eating-dandelions-harvesting-cleaning-and-cooking

Page 64: https://www.organicfacts.net/soba-noodles.html by John Staughton (BASc, BFA) last updated - July 22, 2020

Page 82: https://curejoy.com/content/okra-the-wonder-vegetable-22-the-amazing-health-benefits-of-okra/

Page 107: https://www.drfuhrman.com/blog/186/mighty-mushrooms-boost-immune-function-and-brain-health-and-guard-against-cancer
https://en.wikipedia.org/wiki/Cruciferous_vegetables

Page 164: https://www.hsph.harvard.edu/nutritionsource/food-features/chia-seeds/

Page 181: https://nutritionfacts.org/video/cocoa-good-chocolate-bad/

Page 219: https://draxe.com/nutrition/pomegranate-juice/

RECOMMENDED READING AND WEBSITES

Greger, Michael and Gene Stone. How Not to Die, New York: Flatiron Books, 2015

Kahn, Joel. The Plant-Based Solution. Boulder, CO. Sound True, Inc. 2018

Buettner, Dan. *The Blue Zones: 9 Lessons for Living Longer from people who've lived the longest.* National Geographic; 2012

Campbell, T. Colin and Thomas M. Campbell. *The China Study: The Most Comprehensive Study of Nutrition Ever Conducted and the Starting Implications for Diet, Weight Loss and Long-Term Health.* Dallas, Texas. BenBella Books, 2006

nutritionFacts.org: www.nutritionfacts.org

www.foodrevolution.org

RECIPE INDEX

BY SEASON

BY MEAL CATEGORY

BREAKFAST

BEVERAGES

CONDIMENTS AND MORE

Beverly's Story

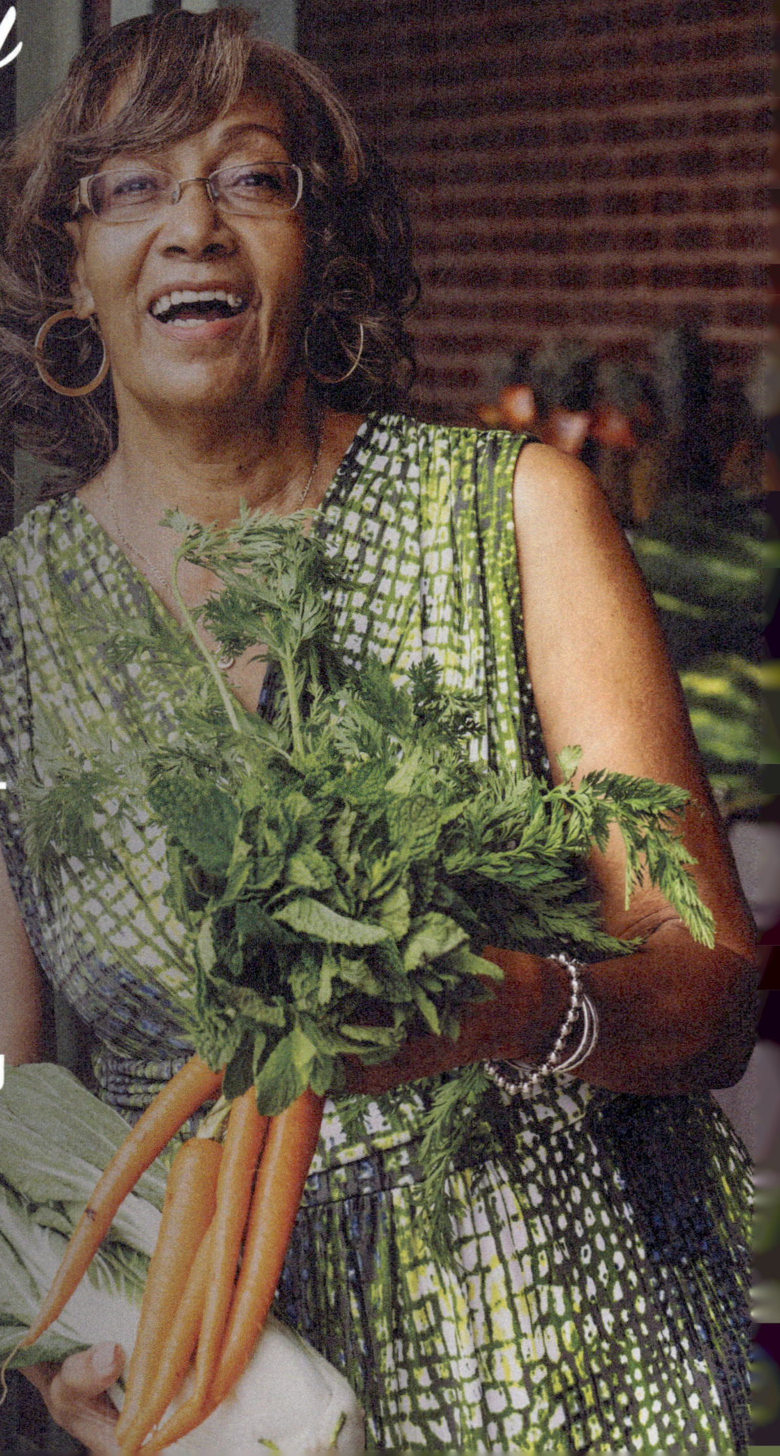

Beverly became interested in healthy eating as a young mother in the early 1970's. The curiosity and fun of learning with other young mothers to make baby food, juice extracting, shopping at the Farmers Market was only the start of a lifelong passion.

Of course, a lot of life has happened in the past 40 year. Life taught Beverly early on that our health and well-being is not one dimensional but a combination of many things. One's intention is key.

Beverly's health journey has been progressive and inspiring through the years. She says, "I never imagined in my lifetime I would see healthy eating – healthy lifestyle celebrated (globally) on the level it currently is". It is very exciting.

Beverly is certified in Plant-Based Nutrition through eCornell. She is the writer and photographer of her blog, Organize Eating. com. Having earned a certificate as a Culinary Community Educator, through Whole Cities Foundation, Beverly presents on topics which also include organizing to be effective.